The HeartSmart Shopper

Nutrition on the Run

Ramona Josephson RDN

Registered Dietitian and Nutritionist

Health Check™ HEART AND STROKE FOUNDATION

Douglas & McIntyre
Vancouver/Toronto

HEART AND STROKE FOUNDATION OF CANADA

97 98 99 00 01 5 4 3 2 1

Douglas & McIntyre
1615 Venables Street
Vancouver, British Columbia
V5L 2H1

Canadian Cataloguing in Publication Data

Josephson, Ramona
The heartsmart shopper

ISBN 1-55054-552-3

1. Nutrition. 2. Grocery shopping. 3. Low-fat diet. 1. Title. II. Title: The heart smart shopper.
TX356.J67 1997 613.2 C97-910396-7

Editing by Elizabeth Wilson
Writing support by Angela Murrills
Cover and text design by DesignGeist
Illustrations by Michela Sorrentino Design
Printed and bound in Canada by Best Book Manufacturers
Printed on acid-free paper

The publisher gratefully acknowledges the assistance of the Canada Council for the Arts and of the British Columbia Ministry of Tourism, Small Business and Culture.

Contents

Foreword

As the Chair of the National Health Promotion Committee of the Heart and Stroke Foundation of Canada, I have had the distinct pleasure of being involved with the Foundation as it increasingly promotes the direct relationship of nutrition to healthy living for all Canadians. The Foundation's momentum in this area has been significant, from the research of the early 1980s to the many HeartSmart™ cookbooks, restaurant programs, cooking courses, videos and other community activities.

The Heart and Stroke Foundation is now on the eve of launching its Health Check™ program, which will change forever the way Canadians choose food products for a healthy diet. The Health Check™ program, developed and administered by the Heart and Stroke Foundation, is a not-for-profit, on-pack program whereby food producers offer their products/formulas for nutritional analysis by pre-set standards. If a product meets the program's criteria, the producer may apply to display a Health Check™ logo on the package, in conjunction with nutrition information and a helpful message for consumers.

For many years, Canadian consumers have tried to apply the principles of Canada's Food Guide to Healthy Eating while shopping. The Health Check™ program, as it unfolds across a wide spectrum of grocery products, will provide a new relevance to these nutrition principles by bringing them to life—right on the product packaging.

Ramona Josephson's creative and practical book is empathetic to the hectic and over-committed lives that so many of us lead. Together with the Health Check™ program, *The HeartSmart Shopper* will empower you to make healthy food choices in the supermarket. Her book is full of simple icons and visual cues, which are exactly what so many Canadians have requested: tools to assist them in healthy grocery shopping. After reading this, I am sure you will see your shopping cart in an entirely new light!

Bretta Maloff

Bretta Maloff, M.Ed., R.D.
Volunteer Chair
National Health Promotion Committee

Preface

For the past 40 years, public support of the Heart and Stroke Foundation of Canada has enabled us to be the leader in heart disease and stroke research investment in Canada. Constantly in search of results that could make a difference to patients, people at risk and the general public, the Foundation has produced a wide range of materials and programs that empower you to make heart-healthy choices.

We know that small, everyday changes can make a big difference to your health outcomes, yet sometimes it seems so hard to know where to start. *The HeartSmart Shopper: Nutrition on the Run* begins in a very practical place: choosing your food in the supermarket. Author and nutritionist Ramona Josephson bases this book on the precepts of Canada's Food Guide to Healthy Eating and helps you use your shopping cart as a nutritional barometer in an unforgettable way. The book's illustrations transform sound nutrition into sensible and memorable bits of information. Ramona's Fat Budgeting guidelines throughout the book are reassuringly tangible in their use of the old-fashioned teaspoon, making it easier than ever to choose healthy alternatives.

In addition, *The HeartSmart Shopper* showcases another milestone in the Foundation's history: the launching of our new food information Health Check™ program. As the program rolls out across a wide spectrum of products, the Health Check™ on-pack symbol will become a concrete guide to making healthy choices right in the supermarket. It is a not-for-profit program, developed and administered by the Heart and Stroke Foundation of Canada.

An altogether unique nutrition journey is about to begin—and we are delighted to have you along!

Gary Sutherland

Gary Sutherland
Volunteer President
Heart and Stroke Foundation of Canada

The Health Check™ Program

Since it's inception 40 years ago, the Heart and Stroke Foundation of Canada and indeed, comparable organizations around the world, have turned research into practice by encouraging people to adopt healthy lifestyle practices—especially when it comes to eating. Through its many HeartSmart™ programs, the Foundation has long promoted awareness of the relationship of nutrition to the risk factors for heart disease and stroke. Over the last eight years, the Foundation's growing list of HeartSmart™ cookbooks has sold over 1.5 million copies!

The Foundation is now preparing to implement its revolutionary Health Check™ program, a comprehensive food and nutrition information program based on nutrient criteria for total health. As a not-for-profit initiative of the Heart and Stroke Foundation of Canada, the program will be administered independently of the food industry.

The Health Check™ program has been set up as a self–supporting initiative on a cost–recovery basis through levies paid by manufacturers. The program was developed in response to Canadian consumers' demands for more nutrition information. Research shows that the majority of Canadian consumers are concerned about what you and your families eat; over half of you are very concerned. Canadians believe that nutrition is an important determinant of your health, and you apply this belief to your eating habits. According to a 1995 survey by the Canadian Council of Grocery Distributors and Food Marketing Institute, one in five consumers recently changed his or her eating habits in response to nutritional concerns.

In a 1997 Heart and Stroke Foundation Health Information Study, 83 per cent of consumers identified food package labels as a place they would find valuable as a source of information on healthy eating. Consumers ranked nutrition labelling as one of three top priorities for the grocery industry, yet your satisfaction with the amount of information on food labels has declined since 1991. A 1996 study by the Food and Consumer Product Manufacturers of Canada found that consumers report having "real trouble" reading product labels and understanding nutrition terms. With our increasingly hectic and stressful lives, the time to read complex food labels in the supermarket just isn't there!

The Heart and Stroke Foundation of Canada has a long history of leadership in nutrition issues in Canada. Now the Health Check™ program will give Canadians additional tools and the support you need to make wise food choices when grocery shopping. The program presents itself to the shopper as a logo and explanatory message, combined with a nutrition information panel on each participating product. No more confusion!

The National Heart Foundation of Australia has operated a similar program for the past eight years, as has the American Heart Association for the past two years. Both programs have found huge acceptance by consumers and industry alike. Here in Canada, the Heart and Stroke Foundation's Health Check™ program is being developed under the direction of a National Technical Advisory Committee, with ongoing consultation with appropriate federal government departments and a number of national stakeholders with an interest in nutrition issues.

The focus of the Health Check™ program is general healthy eating (not only heart-healthy eating) evaluated within the context of a total diet (not only on a product by product basis). The program's nutritional criteria are consistent with those that underpin Canada's Food Guide to Healthy Eating and are founded on the central tenets of total health—the idea that all foods can fit in a healthy diet.

The program is voluntary. Manufacturers submit their products for review against published nutritional criteria for appropriate food categories. A product's fat, fibre, calcium, starch, sodium, vitamin and mineral levels are evaluated as required. If the product meets the criteria and the manufacturer applies for its inclusion to the program, they are licensed, remit a levy to the Heart and Stroke Foundation and display the Health Check™ logo and message on their package. To preserve the program's integrity, random checks of participating products will be conducted independently.

Due to the program's voluntary and phased-in nature, it may take a few years for Health Check™ to become a comprehensive guide to food choices. As the program grows, both with more participants and across a widening number of food categories, the Heart and Stroke Foundation of Canada will invest in a broad health promotion program and nutrition research with the specific goal of increasing awareness among Canadians about wise food choices and general healthy eating. Watch for the Health Check™ program in the months ahead, and visit the Internet website at http://www.healthcheck.org.

The Heart and Stroke Foundation of Canada

Author's Acknowledgements

Being a professional dietitian and nutrition consultant has its occupational hazards! I find myself bombarded with questions on nutrition in arenas that extend far beyond my counselling office—the gym, the supermarket, by the media ... However, the questions keep me on my toes, and I learn the issues on people's minds.

The HeartSmart Shopper was written with the love and support of my husband, Ken Karasick, and my teens, who encouraged me to, "Just keep writing as if you were talking to us!" I am delighted when my son, Marc, asks at dinner, "Where's the greens, Mom?" or when my daughter, Jaclyn, drinks milk, "For my bones, Mom." I realize that eventually the messages get through, even in the subtlest of ways.

I would like to thank the following people who contributed their professional expertise, enthusiasm and creativity to the book. From the Heart and Stroke Foundation of Canada: Doug McQuarrie, Director, Health Promotion; Carol Dombrow, consultant Registered Dietitian; and the Health Promotion Initiative Review Committee and staff. From the Heart and Stroke Foundation of B.C. and Yukon: Richard Rees, Executive Director; Fiona Ahrens, Director, Marketing and Communications; and Ursula Fradera and Heather Preece, Registered Dietitians. My creative team included: Angela Murrills, writing support; Michela Sorrentino, illustrations; Sigrid Albert, Gabi Proctor and Catherine Jordan, cover and text design; and Elizabeth Wilson, editing. This book reflects the spirit and inspiration that went into it—fun, coordinated and user-friendly.

The hardest group to satisfy is one's peers—and I put mine to the test, asking many of them to review parts or all of the book. Thanks to my colleagues for your detailed analysis of the contents: Carol Dombrow, Bretta Maloff, consultants to the Heart and Stroke Foundation; Frances Johnson and Shauna Ratner (Healthy Heart Program, St. Paul's Hospital); Donna Forsyth (Children's and Women's Health Centre of B.C.), and Susan Firus (Dial-a-Dietitian of B.C.).

And, of course, thanks to Scott McIntyre of Douglas & McIntyre for acknowledging the value of HeartSmart nutrition and agreeing to publish the book.

INTRODUCTION

Nutrition on the Run

We live in a world of too much choice! So many claims. So many enticing products competing for us to *Buy Me!* Most of us want to give thoughtful consideration to what we're eating, but how do we make intelligent choices when we're on the run?

In *The HeartSmart Shopper*, I'll introduce you to a whole new way of "shopping cart" shopping, with a concept so simple that once it's stamped in your mind it will come alive whenever you go to the store. You'll discover a system of memorable visual symbols that will highlight HeartSmart and All-Star Tips, answer frequently asked questions and offer Penny Wise suggestions. I will show you how to budget fat so easily that you can finally take charge of your choices. Finally, I'll bring your shopping-cart smarts into the kitchen with fun, simple meals that have been family-tested for years in at least one person's kitchen—mine! No complicated recipes, just delicious combinations that you can build on and adapt.

As a nutrition and health educator, I have always looked for innovative ways to take sometimes-complex nutrition issues and make them fun, easy to understand and practical. This zest is reflected in the way I approach everything I do—my nutrition counselling practice, the range of interactive health awareness programs I've developed and my past role as Chief Dietitian of Shaughnessy Hospital and Grace Hospital in Vancouver.

The Heart and Stroke Foundation is determined to reach out to Canadians to empower them to make wise nutrition choices. My task was to take the best of my experience, to hold on to the core values of Canada's Food Guide to Healthy Eating and to convert the volumes of encyclopedic nutrition "stuff" into simple and memorable messages. *The HeartSmart Shopper* does it!

Research has shown that making simple everyday heart-healthy choices *can* make a difference to your health. Whether you're just being introduced to nutrition concepts or you're already a conscientious consumer, this little book may be the greatest investment you've ever made towards your own and your family's health.

Shopping the new shopping-cart way is so simple it will become second nature. I hope you'll have fun as you play with the concepts, trust your own judgment and learn to enjoy all foods in balance.

Ramona Josephson

RDN B.Sc. Hons. Dip. Ther. Diet.

DAILY B.R.E.A.D.

Too hard to remember heart health risk factors? Not with this daily slice of B.R.E.A.D.

B **Blood Pressure and Blood Cholesterol** Do you know your numbers? High blood pressure and high blood cholesterol are risk factors for heart disease and stroke. They are silent conditions—but can be controlled by healthy living and/or by medication.

R **Relaxation** Have you stopped to smell the roses today? Let's face it, our harried lives leave much to be desired. It's not the stress that's the problem—today that's a given. It's how we deal with it that counts. Stress is a risk factor for heart disease, so take a few moments to breathe deeply and relax.

E **Eating Well** Do you? Obesity is a risk factor for heart disease. And most Canadians eat more fat and less fibre than is desirable. It's not for lack of choice. We're surrounded by choices—to buy, prepare and enjoy heart-healthy foods. It's about balance. The wise choice is yours for the taking.

A **Active Living** Are you moving? Activity is a prescription for an endless array of healthy outcomes. It decreases your risk for heart disease, reduces blood pressure and stress levels, helps you manage your weight, and makes you feel great. So remember, every day, to move a little, and then to move a little more.

D **Don't Smoke** A pack-a-day smoker has *twice* the risk for heart disease and stroke as a nonsmoker. And imagine this—each cigarette burns for 12 minutes, and during that time the smoker inhales for a mere 30 seconds. Meanwhile, chemicals are given off into the air and many are known causes of cancer. This is what nonsmokers breathe. So if you do, think D—Don't smoke! For all our sakes.

Make every day another healthy slice of life

SYMBOLS MAKE IT SIMPLE

These simple symbols add up to a recipe for HeartSmart nutrition.

Reading a book on nutrition can be like eating a 12-course dinner without a break. You get indigestion! That's why I've broken the information down into bite-sized pieces and highlighted them with a system of icons—symbols—that help to make each point memorable and simple to use. All together, they add up to a recipe for HeartSmart nutrition.

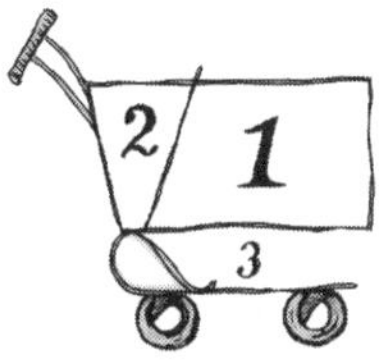

Here's the central concept of this book; it's the express lane to sensible nutrition. Starting page 6, you'll learn to separate your shopping cart into 1-2-3 parts and remember which food groups belong where. When you've got the idea you'll discover it's fun and easy. As the Health Check™ program grows (see page vi), food choices will become even easier—and you'll become a HeartSmart shopper for life.

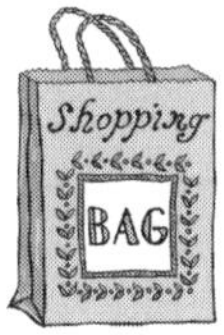

Find out how to shop for vitamins and minerals by choosing foods high in these nutrients.

HeartSmart Tip

These are simple and heart-healthy ways to modify your daily diet to make it HeartSmart. The term HeartSmart incorporates the fat, fibre and sodium guidelines adopted by the Heart and Stroke Foundation that reflect Health Canada's Nutrition Recommendations and Canada's Food Guide to Healthy Eating. A HeartSmart idea always meets these standards, whether as a nutrition tip in this book or a recipe in the highly acclaimed cookbooks from the Heart and Stroke Foundation: *The Lighthearted Cookbook, Lighthearted Everyday Cooking, Simply HeartSmart Cooking, More HeartSmart Cooking,* and *HeartSmart Chinese Cooking.*

Using the teaspoon solution, you'll find out how to make smart fat-budgeting decisions for yourself and your family as you whiz through the supermarket. Just remember, one teaspoon of fat = approximately 5 grams.

These are quick and easy tips to use on a daily basis to boost nutrition—and make *you* a star!

Discover interesting tidbits of information about the foods we eat, food trends and food history. Great to share with friends and family.

Confused about nutrition? I've tried to answer the most common questions. You can also check the Appendix or ask the Heart and Stroke Foundation.

Here you'll find old-fashioned frugality. Find out how to get the most nutrition for your money by following these foolproof buying, storing and cooking tips.

Simple tips about nutritious foods that kids will love—and you'll feel good about giving them. Great ideas for grown-ups too.

This growing not-for-profit food information program from the Heart and Stroke Foundation of Canada will make wise food choices even easier. A Health Check™ logo on the pack tells you that the product has been assessed independently of the food industry against established criteria and is in compliance. See page vi for details.

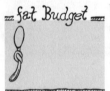

NUTRITION 1-2-3

Organize your shopping cart the way Canada's Food Guide to Healthy Eating organizes food groups for good nutrition.

In the next few pages, I'll show you how to shop nutritiously for the rest of your life. Honest!

One simple idea. Organize your shopping cart the same way that Canada's Food Guide to Healthy Eating organizes food groups for good nutrition. That's it! Sound too easy? Read on.

Nutrition 101 made super simple

The foods we eat contain over 50 different nutrients, each with a story to tell. It seems impossible to remember them all.

Canada's Food Guide to Healthy Eating cuts through the clutter. It's been designed by experts who've spent hours poring over technical literature to structure a diet that will help us stay healthy. The guide groups foods that contain similar, but not identical nutrients, and places them on the bands of the familiar rainbow to illustrate how much of each group we should choose.

According to Canada's Food Guide to Healthy Eating:

The key to good nutrition is to balance a variety of foods from each group and consume them in the appropriate quantities. How do we do that?

- Make more choices from the two outer bands of the rainbow: the grain products, vegetables and fruit.
- Make fewer choices from the two inner bands of the rainbow: the milk products and the meat and alternatives.
- Be cautious about our choices from the foods not listed on the rainbow: the fats, oils and others. These also fit, but remember, it's all about balance.

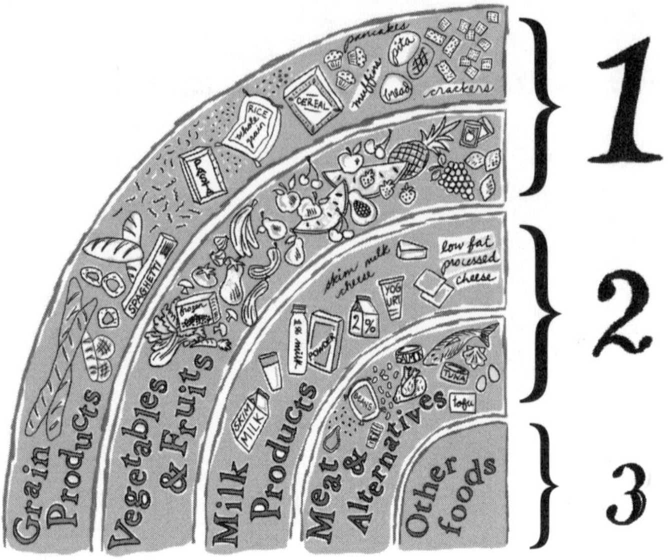

Introducing (tah-dah!) The HeartSmart Shopping Cart

The rainbow is handy, but it's even simpler and more practical to use a universal food guide: the shopping cart. You see it every time you go to the store. I want you to see it now in a totally different way, so that by the end of this book your shopping cart will become the guide to your nutrition choices. It's that simple.

Easy as 1-2-3

Your shopping cart has three parts:

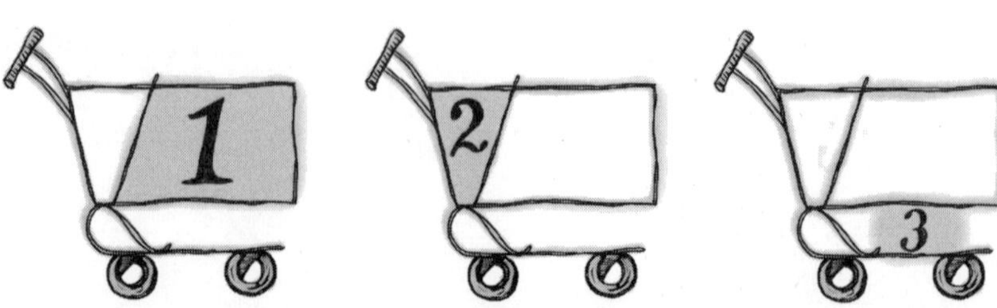

Let your cart be your guide

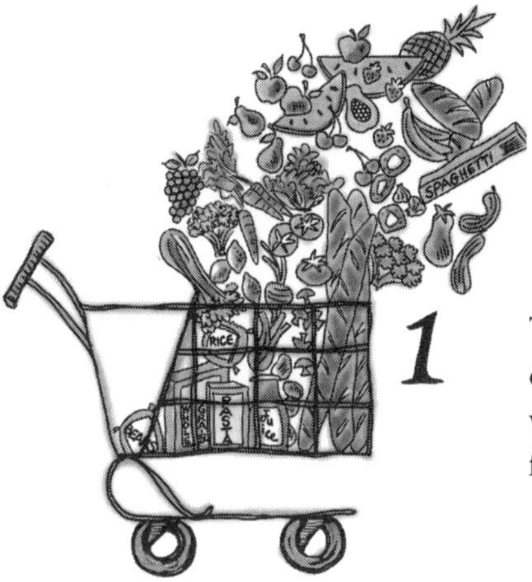

Think Big. Think the two outer bands of the rainbow. Pick grain products, vegetables and fruit in abundance to fill the big part of your cart.

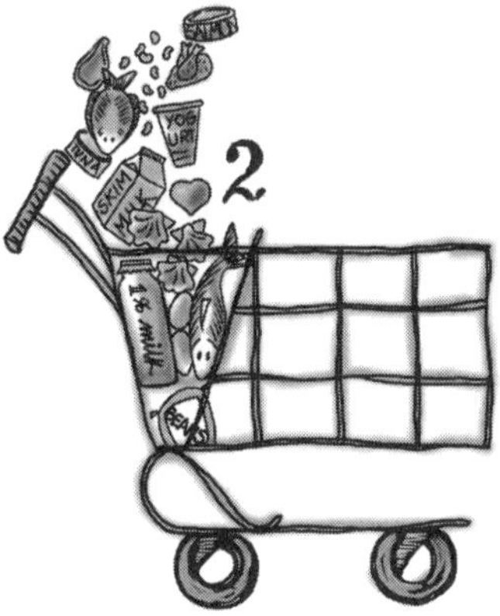

Think Smaller. Think the two inner bands of the rainbow. Use the #2 part to help you choose milk products, meat and alternatives more deliberately.

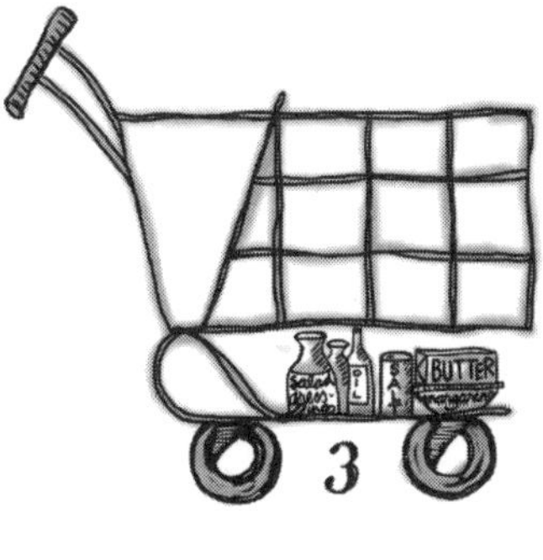

Think Lower. Select your fats, oils and others carefully and put them here.

Nutrition 201

Why choose plant foods in abundance

- Foods from plants are mostly made up of the complex carbohydrates and fibre that our bodies need.
- They contain so little fat that you can forget about it, apart from olives, avocado and coconut.
- They contain no dietary cholesterol.
- They're loaded with vitamins and minerals.

So go ahead! Fill the big #1 part of your cart to your heart's content. Load it up with high-fibre cereals, breads, grains, veggies and fruit.

ALL STAR TIP

Plants are our main source of fibre, and experts recommend that we increase the amount of fibre that we eat. Fibre helps keep us regular, may help prevent bowel diseases and has been connected with the prevention of heart disease, diabetes and some cancers. For more information, see page 28.

QA

Why aren't legumes in this part of the cart?

They could be. Legumes—dried peas, beans and lentils—are like their plant friends. They are low in fat (except soybeans), contain no cholesterol and are high in fibre. No need to limit these! Canada's Food Guide to Healthy Eating places them with meat and alternatives because they are high in protein.

ALL STAR TIP

Meats contain *no* fibre. Fibre is found *only* in plant cells.

Plants contain *no* dietary cholesterol. Cholesterol is found *only* in animal cells.

Why be deliberate with animal foods

The two inner bands of the rainbow contain mostly foods that come directly or indirectly from animals and seafood. Milk products, meat, fish and shellfish belong here. These foods are clustered together because they all provide protein. Many are sources of iron—in a form more readily absorbed than from plant foods—and calcium, zinc and vitamin B12.

But they all contain dietary cholesterol and many contain fat—and often saturated fat—both of which we should try to reduce in our diets.

You'll learn how to make healthy lower-fat choices and to enjoy these foods in moderation. Be deliberate about how you fill the smaller #2 part of your cart, choosing lower-fat milk products, leaner meat, fish and legumes—an easy way to stay within your fat budget.

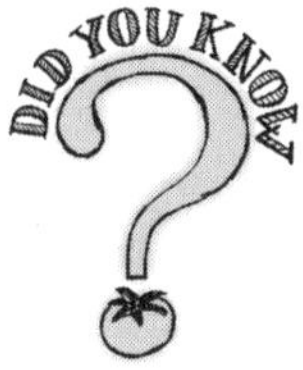

There is *no* single food that contains fibre *and* cholesterol.

Why choose fats, oils and others...carefully

Fats and oils are an integral part of our diet, but most of us eat too much or have trouble making wise choices. Many of the foods they are added to are not on the rainbow because they don't offer enough nutritional value relative to their high fat content.

Keeping this "lower" group in balance can be our biggest challenge. You will find out how to separate the issues of quantity and quality of fats and oils, so that you can think carefully about what you add to the lower part of your cart. Aim to keep quantities small.

- Moms and dads...is the #2 part of the cart where you place your child? A shopping basket in the #1 part should do the trick!
- Psst...placing a shopping basket under your cart will prevent #3 items falling off, and remind you to "contain" what you're buying.

The keys to healthy living

- Enjoy a variety of foods.
- Emphasize high-fibre cereals, breads, other grain products, vegetables and fruit.
- Choose lower-fat dairy products, leaner meats and foods prepared with little or no fat.
- Achieve and maintain a healthy body weight by enjoying regular physical activity and healthy eating.
- Limit salt, alcohol and caffeine.

Source: *Canada's Guidelines for Healthy Eating*

Top **nutrition** at top **speed**

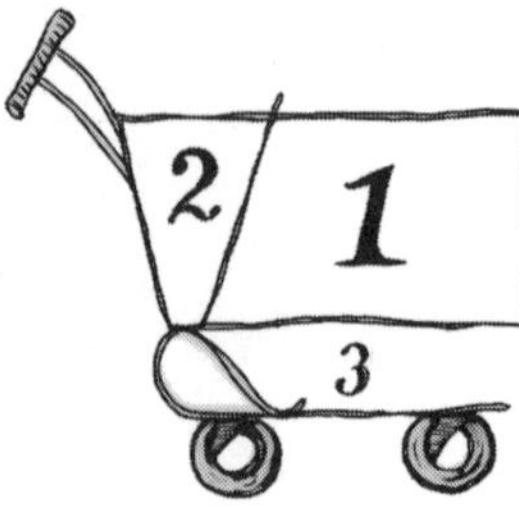

1. Feel free to fill the big #1 part of your cart, loading it up with grains, veggies and fruit.
2. Be deliberate about how you fill the small #2 part of your cart, choosing lower-fat milk products, lean meat, fish and legumes.
3. Think carefully about everything you add to the #3 lower part of your cart.

THE HEARTSMART SHOPPING LIST

Write your shopping list the same way you fill the parts of your cart and you'll provide your family with variety and balance.

Grab a piece of paper and imagine it's divided into three unequal parts. Fold the page in half from top to bottom. Open it out and then fold the bottom half in to a third of its depth. Write #1, #2 and #3 on the three sections like this:

1 Big! Load up—with grains, vegetables and fruit.

2 Smaller! Be deliberate—choose lower-fat milk products, leaner meats, fish and legumes.

3 Lower! Think carefully—limit fats, oils and others.

As you write down what you plan to buy, you reinforce your nutrition savvy by allocating those foods to the #1, #2 and #3 parts of your list because the list reflects the way you fill your shopping cart.

After you've written your list, ask yourself, *Have I included enough whole grains, veggies and fruit? Did I choose lower-fat milk products, and are there enough of them? Did I select a range of lower-fat meats, fish and legumes?* Last of all ask yourself, *Did I think carefully about fats, oils and others—are there too many?* Maybe you'll need to revise your list.

With this list in your hand, you'll whiz through the aisles, secure in the knowledge that even on the run you're a HeartSmart shopper.

- **Avoid going to the store when you're hungry. If you've got the growlies, it's all too easy to make impulsive choices and throw away your fat budget.**
- **Leave your shopping list on the fridge. As you and your family add to it, you'll reinforce the importance of the food groups and how to establish healthy, balanced eating habits.**

FAT BUDGETING MADE EASY

Here's a simple technique to budget your fat intake—the teaspoon solution.

It's no secret—we're eating too much fat. Canada's Food Guide to Healthy Eating and the Heart and Stroke Foundation recommend that we reduce our fat intake in total, and be more particular about what kind of fat we eat. We need to separate the fat issue into:

Fat 101— Quantity Fat 201— Quality.

A little fat is OK. In fact it's not just OK, it's necessary. The problem is, most of us eat too much. After 1919 our daily intake shot up from 27% to 40% of our daily calories. Wow! It's fortunately on the downturn now and currently hovers around 36% to 38%. Most experts consider that the fat in our daily diet should equal no more than 30% OF OUR TOTAL CALORIES daily.

Fat 101—Quantity

All fats are a concentrated source of energy. They supply nine calories per gram—more than twice the energy provided by carbohydrates and protein. Too much fat = increased risk of obesity, heart disease and diabetes. Health experts agree that the food we eat should provide us with no more than 30% of calories from fat. But what does this mean in everyday terms, and how much fat should *you* budget in a day?

The daily fat intake recommended for the average man and woman is represented in the following chart.

	Calories/day	Grams of fat
Women, 19 to 74	1800 – 2000	65 or less
Men, 19 to 74	2300 – 3000	90 or less

This chart shows you how many *grams* of fat you should consume in a day. It's a useful guide if you are in the habit of reading labels or food composition books. But not all foods are labelled, and who has the time to read lists and charts? So what do you do?

I find it easier to remember important concepts by using visual images, so I would like to propose the Teaspoon Solution: a visual way to budget your fat intake for the day.

Fat budget for a day —the good old teaspoon

Here's a way to keep fat budgeting really simple. Visualize a teaspoon of fat. That teaspoon equals approximately 5 grams of fat.

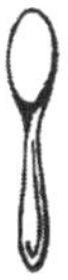

1 tsp. fat = approximately 5 grams of fat

Each time you sit down to eat a meal or snack, visualize the teaspoons of fat contained in what you are about to eat. Throughout this book, I have listed approximately how many teaspoons of fat are in many of the foods we eat. These are average amounts and are a useful guide to making HeartSmart decisions. Now, use the handy chart that follows to determine how many of those teaspoons you should budget in a day.

	Calories/day	Grams of fat	Teaspoons of Fat
Women, 19 to 74	1800 – 2000	65 or less	13 or less
Men, 19 to 74	2300 – 3000	90 or less	18 or less

As you use up your fat budget throughout the day, visualize how many teaspoons remain. When you shop, use the fat budget lists at the beginning of each chapter and make a mental note of the teaspoons of fat in your favourite foods choices. You may be surprised by how many lower-fat options you have. All foods can fit—enjoy the variety and decide for yourself how to spend your teaspoons of fat.

QA

What about my Personal Fat Budget?
A person's fat budget and calorie requirement are dependent on their level of physical activity. To calculate your personal fat budget, refer to My Four Steps to Estimating Your Personal Fat Budget on page 125.

ALL STAR TIP

- Some foods you buy are labelled with the fat represented in grams. Remember: *5 grams of fat = approximately 1 teaspoon fat.* Divide the grams by 5 and you can see, as a general guideline, where a food fits into your fat-budgeting chart.
- Look for the Health Check™ logo on a growing number of food packages. Products that carry the Health Check™ logo are wise choices based on Canada's Food Guide to Healthy Eating.

KIDSTUFF

These fat budget goals don't apply to children who are still growing. Children often need the calories of higher-fat foods to help them develop. Fat should be reduced gradually so that by the time they end puberty their fat intake is that of an adult. In the meantime, let them learn by example—yours—how to enjoy lower-fat foods.

DID YOU KNOW

While you should try to consume no more than 30% of your calories from fat, you don't need to relate the 30% value to every individual food to see if it fits (see page 127). The 30% figure applies to your overall diet—what you eat daily or even weekly. Using the fat budget system you can balance lower-fat foods with higher-fat foods to meet your goal. A HeartSmart diet doesn't mean cutting fat out. It just means cutting down—and choosing foods carefully.

HeartSmart Tip

It's not *only* the quantity of fat, it's the quality. Look for HeartSmart tips in each part of your cart.

Fat 201—Quality

Screech! Put the brakes on! Fat can be saturated, monounsaturated, polyunsaturated, hydrogenated or a trans fatty acid. What do they mean?? And how can a HeartSmart shopper make sense of them on the run? Read on . . .

Not all fats are created equal

Saturated, monounsaturated and polyunsaturated fats (see Appendix, page 126, for definitions) appear in different combinations in different foods. So for instance, when we say that foods from animal sources contain saturated fats, it's not actually the whole story. In fact, they contain *mostly* saturated fatty acids. Try to choose foods that contain the *lower* amounts of saturated fatty acids.

Saturated fat AND hydrogenated fat are the ones to reduce

Saturated fat is found naturally in many foods, but is also manufactured when unsaturated fat is processed. This is called hydrogenation, a process used to change liquid oils into a spread or solid form. Be on the alert for this word on food packaging labels. These fats raise blood cholesterol, so you should eat less of them.

Here's where you'll most often find saturated fat

- In the #2 part of your cart: milk products and many meat products are high in saturated fats. This is why you need to budget fat wisely here.
- In the #3 part of your cart: the tropical vegetable oils—palm, palm kernel and coconut oil, often used in food processing—are high in saturated fat. You'll see these names listed on the label in the ingredient list. The less you choose the better.

Here's where you'll most often find hydrogenated fats

- In the #1 part of your cart: many baked goods use hydrogenated fat.
- In the #3 part of your cart: many products contain fats that are processed to harden them. Look out for the words "hydrogenated" or "partially hydrogenated" in the ingredient list and choose these less often.

DID YOU KNOW

When a fat is hydrogenated, the process creates saturated fat as well as trans fatty acids. Both fats raise blood cholesterol. Research into trans fatty acids is relatively new so you won't find these listed on a label. For now, be on the alert when you see the word "hydrogenated" on the ingredient list.

HeartSmart Tip

Non-hydrogenated margarines can be made spreadable without having trans fats. This is done with the addition of a small amount of tropical oil in manufacturing.

ALL STAR TIP

If a label shows the fat breakdown, a little math can help you figure out the trans fatty acids. Add up the three fatty acids (saturated, monounsaturated and polyunsaturated) and subtract from the total fat. Trans fatty acids are what's left—the less the better.

Fat budgeting at a glance

Canada's Food Guide to Healthy Eating divides foods into bands of a rainbow to highlight groups of foods abundant in similar nutrients. However, some foods have too much fat relative to their nutritional content. Use the fat budget chart at the beginning of each "shopping cart" chapter to decide how to spend your fat budget to suit your needs.

SUPERMARKET SAVVY

Every choice you make, every old habit you break, can make a big difference to your family's health in the long run.

The grocery store doors slide apart and suddenly you're in a world of amazing foodstuffs and alluring choices. New products, exotic fruits and vegetables, different cuts of meat, seafood and shellfish that you may never have seen before, herbs and seasonings from the world's four corners. Enticing signage and labels that shout *Buy Me!* All the opportunities you could imagine to make fabulous meals—and to tempt you away from HeartSmart nutrition. So where do you begin? How do you stay nutrition smart . . . on the run?

Filling a HeartSmart shopping cart can start with a research trip. Once you've read through this book, investing a single half hour can pay lifelong dividends in terms of good nutrition.

I know, I know—it isn't the most exciting invitation you've ever had. But taking a new look at nutrition means looking at your supermarket in a different light.

There are over 25,000 items to choose from in large supermarkets. Each time you walk into one you have hundreds of decisions to make. And yet the average shopper usually takes just seconds to decide what to buy. Doing a little research during a quiet time at your usual store can help you shop just as quickly, but far more wisely.

Go through this book at home. I've tried to keep it simple because I want you to remember a few simple facts. Then put theory into practice at your supermarket. The first time, don't buy a single thing! Just go from aisle to aisle, look at your family's favourites and recall what you've read. After just this one research trip to the supermarket, you'll be amazed at how fast you can select wisely, and be nutrition and money wise!

Run each item through your nutrition scanner

Does it fit with what you're trying to achieve? Will it help you keep to your fat budget? Compared with similar products on the shelf, how does it stack up? Does it have more fat and salt than other nutrients? Soon you'll be answering these questions automatically as you make the best choices and tick off your shopping list.

Every time you buy your groceries, you're investing in your family's long-term health. This is serious stuff. Every choice you make, every old habit you break can make a big difference to their health and yours in the long run.

Going eyeball to eyeball with the products on the shelf

Items that are displayed from the waist to eye level and above sell more. In fact, this is the most desirable space on the supermarket shelves. When you look below you will often find bargains and better deals. Adult cereals (such as the high-fibre ones) are placed on the top shelves. Kids' cereals—and other junior favourites such as cookies and fruit snacks—are often placed at your kids' eye level. Basic cereals that may have been on the market for years are often on the bottom shelf.

Why items are where they are

To entice you to buy! Standing in the checkout line is a bore. After you've read about the latest Elvis sighting, there's not much else to do . . . except shop. No wonder supermarkets stock this area with magazines, candies, batteries and other small impulse items.

Usually, the outer ring of the supermarket is where you'll find perishable foods: baked goods, fruits and vegetables, meats and the milk products. Staples, such as milk and eggs, are often right at the back of the store so that even if you're only popping in for some basics you'll find yourself walking by shelves of tempting items. Be careful!

Cross-merchandising means displaying two products together that go together. Salsa and taco chips. Fresh fish and tartar sauce. Lettuces and gourmet salad dressings. Pasta and pasta sauce. Convenient? Yes. But do a mental check as to how they fit into your HeartSmart shopping cart.

New products are often displayed at the end of the aisle because this is where you slow down to turn the corner.

And what can entice you more than the fragrance of the bakery or the smell of free samples?

TAKE A LOOK AT LABELS

Food package labels can be a wealth of information if you know what to look for.

New! Improved! Cholesterol free! No added sugar! Reading labels in the supermarket is the ultimate in window shopping. Labels are designed to attract our attention. They can be a useful tool to help you select foods for healthy eating and to compare products. But while all labels conform to regulations, they can be misinterpreted. Canadian laws are currently under review by Health Canada.

Become an informed label reader. Find out what's in it, what's on it and what's not. Learn to read between the lines to find out what you need to know. There are three components to a product label.

1. The ingredient list

Items are listed in *descending* order by weight. At the top of the list is the ingredient that there's *most* of. At the bottom of the list is the ingredient there's *least* of. This is especially useful to know if you are on a special diet or need to avoid any particular ingredient.

DID YOU KNOW

While ingredients are listed in descending order by weight, manufacturers don't have to say how much of each is used. Comparing products precisely using this list is almost impossible.

ALL STAR TIP

Reading labels can help you get the most value for your money. If two similar products cost the same, but one has more of the key ingredient, it might be a better choice. For instance, apple juice lists apple juice as the first ingredient. Apple drink lists water, sugar and colouring.

How to speak label-ese

Earlier in this book (page iv) you read about the Health Check™ on-pack labelling program which is intended to act as your quick and easy guide to wise product choices. It is a new, expanding program so while more products join up, you will need to read labels at face value. Here's a list of many of the different words for fat, sugar and salt that you'll find on labels.

Fats

- fat, lard, shortening
- hydrogenated vegetable oils
- vegetable oil
- coconut/palm oils, tropical oils
- mono and diglycerides, tallow

Sugars

- sugar, honey, molasses
- dextrose, sucrose, fructose
- maltose, lactose (words that end in -ose)
- dextrin, maltodextrin, invert sugar
- maple syrup, corn syrup, malt syrup

Salts

- salt, MSG
- anything with the word sodium
- baking soda, baking powder, brine
- kelp, soy sauce

Read between the lines

If enriched white flour is the first ingredient on the list, that loaf of bread you're looking at is unlikely to be high in fibre. And those cookies—if oil is at the head of the list of ingredients, it means they're likely to be high in fat. Also remember, sugar may not be listed first on a list of ingredients but it may be there in quantity. The trick is to add up all the sugars listed under other names (see list above).

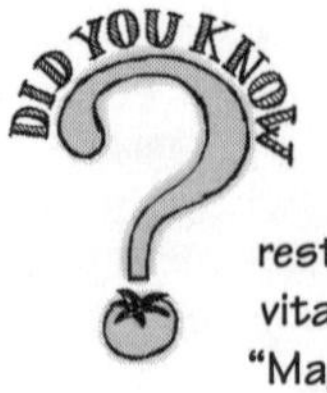

"Fortified" or "enriched" means that nutrients are added or that some of the nutrients lost in processing have been restored. For instance, milk is enriched with vitamins A and D.

"May contain" means an ingredient is optional.

2. The nutrition information panel

This part of the label is at present voluntary for manufacturers. It is here you might find information on calories per serving size, values for fat, carbohydrates, protein, various minerals and vitamins.

Counting calories? Look on the label under "energy" to find how many calories are in a serving. Check whether the serving size is typical for you. If not, adjust.

Cutting down on fat? Look under "total fat" in grams. Use this information to compare brands and to make lower-fat choices.

Want more fibre? Look under "carbohydrates" and choose products with more than 2 grams of fibre.

Cutting back on salt? The less the better.

™HEART AND STROKE FOUNDATION

The new labelling program from the Heart and Stroke Foundation makes the process much simpler. Look for the Health Check™ logo on the packaging and you'll be sure to find a nutrition information panel.

How's your appetite? If you eat half—or double—the serving size shown on the nutrition information panel, remember to halve or double the nutrient values.

3. Nutrition claims

This is the sizzle on the package that can entice you to buy a product—or pass it by. These claims highlight a nutritional feature of a product, and are allowed by Health Canada because they are backed up by facts (see Appendix, page 128). Because so many of us focus on reducing fat and calories, we often read more into these claims than we should. Be sure you don't misinterpret the message.

"Less" or "reduced in fat, calories or salt"

These words mean that the product contains lower quantities of this nutrient or ingredient. This information can be useful when comparing similar products.

Refer to the nutrition information panel (when present) to check out the actual amounts.

"Light" or "lite"

These words are often used to describe a food reduced in fat and energy, e.g., some milk products and salad dressings—but not always. They may simply refer to the taste, colour or texture of a food, as is often true when it refers, for example, to an oil. So, when you see "lite" or "light" on the label, ask yourself, Light in what? before assuming it is low in calories. The answer? Read the fine print on the label.

"Cholesterol free" or "low in saturated fat"

These products may not necessarily be low in fat. Vegetable oils, for example, contain no cholesterol and, while they may be low in saturated fat, they are still 100% fat.

"Fat free"

A product free of fat is not necessarily low in calories. It may still be high in sugar.

"No added sugar"

While it may not have added sugar, a product may still be high in natural sugar.

Contains a "healthy" ingredient such as fibre

Of course fibre is healthy, but watch out for other ingredients such as fat and salt that may cancel out potential benefits. It's about balance again.

"All vegetable oil"

These words do not necessarily mean low in saturated fat. The oil used in a product such as cookies may be hydrogenated (or partially hydrogenated) or it may be a saturated vegetable oil such as palm oil. (See Appendix, page 126.)

"Low calorie"

If a product package reads "low calorie," then you can rest assured that it *is* low in fat *and* sugar, because many products derive their calories from these two sources.

As the Health Check™ program grows, more and more products will display the decal, making wise food choices even easier.

PENNY WISE...ON THE RUN

Careful shopping habits and storage smarts are among the most valuable skills you can acquire.

Gulp! Over 20 years a family of four is estimated to spend well over $100,000 in the supermarket. The good news is that the more you know, the better the food you can buy for your money. Careful shopping habits and storage smarts are among the most valuable skills you can acquire. Literally. Over time you can save thousands of dollars.

Food wasn't always trademarked. In great-grandmother's era all crackers came from the cracker barrel. If customers were dissatisfied the store owner simply bought from another source. Brand names came into being in the 1940s. This way the brand guaranteed quality and the same taste every time. But today no-name brands apply the same consistent quality control standards—and you're not paying the extra cents that subsidize advertising. Your decision.

Six cost cutting tips

1. Store brands can save you a bundle. Often they are the least expensive, because they are not advertised like popular brand names. Is there a difference? Judge for yourself. Compare ingredient lists and read the nutrition information panels if available. Ask your family or friends to taste both products (without telling them which is which) and let them decide.

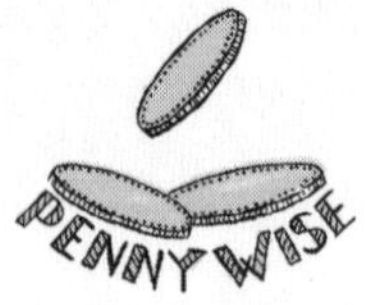

2. Larger doesn't always mean cheaper. Don't always buy the biggest size. Compare the unit price of different sizes of similar items to see if you're really saving money. Check the little tab on the supermarket shelf which displays the price per gram or per millilitre. It's information worth looking at.

3. Buy in bulk...sometimes. Scooping out as much as you need from a bin may not be cheaper, especially if you need to buy large quantities. Sounds silly doesn't it? But in fact, you get more value in "bulk" buying when you only need small quantities. Pre-packaged items are usually more economical for larger purchases. Look for the scales in this section of the supermarket and weigh the amount you buy so you won't be surprised when you get to the check-out.

   Buying warehouse-size packages of cereal is a terrific idea if you have teenagers. You'll never run out and the price is considerably lower too. But that family-size jar of fresh salsa will only be a super buy if you have space to store it and can use it up before the "best before" date.

4. Check local flyers for seasonal foods and weekly specials, but think twice about running around from one store to another to pick up your weekly purchase. Figure out how much time you'll spend. Gas costs too.

   Enjoy seasonal produce for all it's worth—and stash some in the freezer. That way you'll have home-frozen raspberries in the middle of winter for a lot less than the cost of the imported fresh ones.

5. Eat more vegetable proteins. Try peanut butter sandwiches, lentil soup with crackers, baked beans with corn bread or tofu with rice and stir-fried veggies. All offer high-quality nutrition at lower prices.

6. Take the extra time at home to store food wisely to ensure that it doesn't end up in the garbage can. The Penny Wise icon will point you to storage tips for each food group throughout the book.

Section 1 of your shopping cart

Grains

Vegetables and Fruit

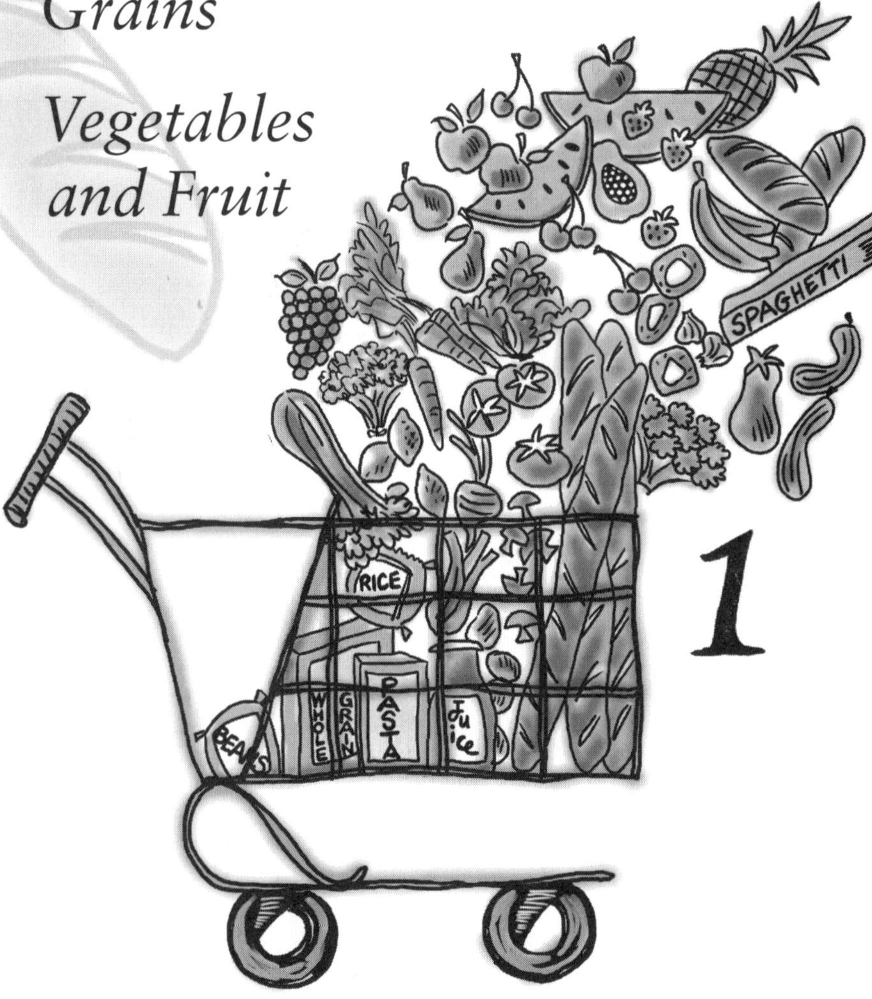

1

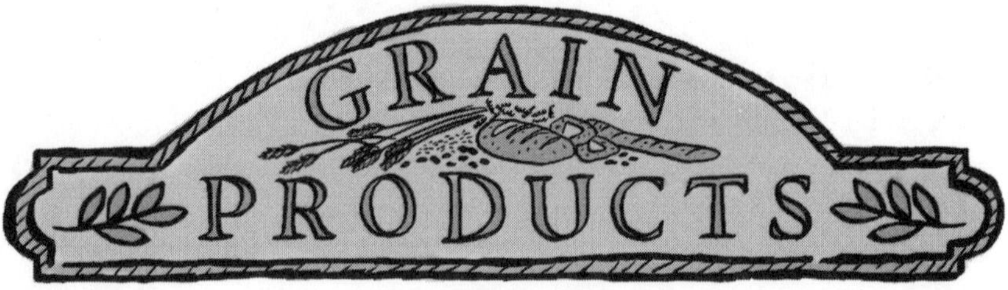

Fill up the big #1 part of your shopping cart—load up on grains.

HeartSmart shoppers, we're on our way. Smell that crusty loaf just out of the oven. Picture a bowl of steaming hot oatmeal on a frosty winter morning. Delicious!

Grains—a small word for the explosion of choices we find in the supermarket. How lucky we are. They're low in fat and they can be loaded with fibre. So feel free to fill the #1 part of your cart with abandon.

Bakery shelves bulge with whole-wheat loaves, buns, bagels, rolls and pitas. Pasta tempts us with all its different shapes. Spaghetti, lasagna, bows, shells and spirals—you could feed your family a different pasta every day of the month. Brown, wild, basmati . . . explore the world of rice. Check out the delicious "new" grains too, like bulgur, quinoa and cornmeal.

Grains are warming in winter and many make tasty main-dish salads. Add a handful of grains to a soup and suddenly soup becomes supper. Making rice? Just add meat or fish and lots of cubed fresh vegetables (a great way to use up leftovers) and you have a meal. And another nice piece of news: Grains aren't only a great way to keep our health on track; they do the same for our fat budget. What's more, they're a bargain.

So grab as much as you like. Pile up the #1 part of your HeartSmart shopping cart with whole-grain products, and eat them more often.

Take five—and more if you can

Canada's Food Guide to Healthy Eating recommends 5 to 12 servings of grains a day. Hard to eat that much? Not a bit.

One serving means:

- 1/2 cup (125 mL) cooked cereal
- 1 slice bread
- 1/2 bagel, pita or bun
- 3/4 cup (175 mL) ready-to-eat cereal
- 1/2 cup (125 mL) pasta or rice (cooked)

Fat budgeting with grain products

Most grains are low in fat. That's why it's so easy to load up the #1 part of your cart. Choose a variety of foods from the grain group to get many important nutrients.

Check the fat budget list and decide how you want to spend your fat budget.

fat Budget

Grain products:

almost 0 tsp. fat	most breads, cereals, rice, pasta and other grains
1 tsp. fat	1 small granola bar 2 medium pancakes 5 soda crackers
2 tsp. fat	1 croissant 1 medium muffin 1 danish pastry 1 plain doughnut
3 tsp. fat	1/2 cup (125 mL) granola 1 cup instant ramen noodles

1 teaspoon fat = approximately 5 grams of fat.
These numbers are averages.

To find out what nutrients grain products offer and where they fit in the total nutrition picture, see Appendix, page 124.

fat Budget

The teaspoons of fat in granola, pastries, muffins, cookies, cake or doughnuts add up fast relative to their nutritional content. Choose these less often.

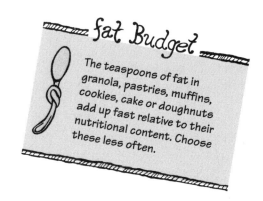

Get fired up about fibre

The more fibre you eat, the easier it is for your intestinal tract to function smoothly. The easier it is to maintain a healthy weight too. Eating carbohydrates helps you cut back on calorie-dense fats and sweets. Research shows that fibre may help to prevent certain forms of cancer and lower our cholesterol. We used to think fibre was useless. Big mistake. Now we know just how important it really is.

Fibre is a type of carbohydrate found only in plants. It's a special component of food that isn't absorbed. Instead, it passes right through your system. There are two types—soluble and insoluble.

Soluble fibre can help control blood sugar. It can also help lower blood cholesterol especially if it is high.

Best sources of soluble fibre:
- Oat bran
- Oatmeal
- Legumes (dried beans, peas and lentils)
- Pectin-rich fruits (apples, strawberries, citrus fruits)

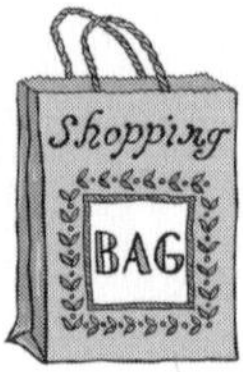

Insoluble fibre helps to prevent and control bowel problems and may be important in the prevention of certain cancers.

Best sources of insoluble fibre:
- Wheat bran and wheat bran cereals
- Whole-grain foods like whole-wheat bread
- Fruit and vegetables including skins and seeds when practical

Double your fibre! The typical North American diet contains about 12 to 15 grams of dietary fibre. Most authorities recommend aiming for 25 to 35 grams. Here's how:
- Fibre-rich cereal for breakfast
- Raisins, banana or orange slices on your cereal
- Low-fat bran or oatmeal muffin
- Whole-grain breads
- Tons of veggies and fruit for snacks
- Beans, peas and lentils
- High-fibre cereal on casseroles

Suddenly increasing your fibre may leave you feeling bloated. Up your fibre intake gradually and be sure to drink 6 to 8 cups (1.5 to 2 litres) of water daily.

HeartSmart Tip Many products contain fibre—but how much? Reading the fine print will tell you.

If the package says:	It means this much fibre per serving:
"A source of dietary fibre"	at least 2 grams
"High source of dietary fibre"	at least 4 grams
"Very high source of dietary fibre"	at least 6 grams

A trip down the bakery aisle

Bagels, baguettes, French and Italian peasant breads, pita, pumpernickel, rye, English muffins, tortillas . . . can you believe the number of breads we have available? Bread can be a powerhouse of nutrition. It supplies a large part of our daily carbohydrate intake. It's also a good source of fibre, thiamin, riboflavin, niacin, iron and trace minerals.

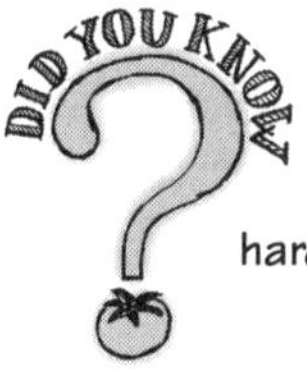

One slice of most breads provides only 70 calories and hardly any fat.

fat Budget

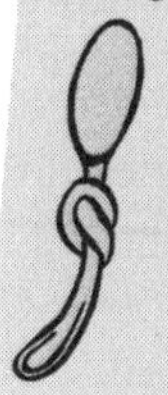

One croissant supplies 2 teaspoons of fat. Choose a bun or bagel instead to help your fat budget.

Is today's bread better bred? Not necessarily.

Great-grandmother had no choice. She had to serve bread made from stone-ground flour. Little did she know how healthy it was. Back then, only the inedible husk was removed when the miller ground the flour. As the wheat was ground between two stones, the husks were sifted or blown out. What was left was packed with nutrients. Along came modern times—and machinery that could get rid of not only the husk but also nutrient-rich wheat germ and high-fibre bran. All that was left was the smooth, white endosperm. White bread became a status symbol. Crunchy brown bread made from nutritious whole-grain flour was considered old-fashioned.

Then problems developed. Many people began to develop deficiencies of iron and the B vitamins, niacin, thiamin and riboflavin. An Enrichment

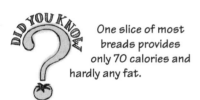

Act was passed in 1942 stating that these four nutrients must be added back to refined flour. This law is still in effect and so, whatever their colour, grain products, breads and cereals manufactured in Canada have been enriched with at least these four nutrients. Folate is now being added too.

But it's still not as nutritious as the original wheat grain. Many of the nutrients found in the whole grain—magnesium, zinc, vitamin B6, vitamin E, chromium and fibre—are lost in white bread.

Bread buying made easy

Whole-wheat flour, wheat bread, cracked wheat … which to choose?

- For nutritious high-fibre bread, look for the word *whole* grain, e.g., *whole wheat*, in the ingredient list. Wheat *bran* boosts the fibre content. Remember: the first ingredient on the list is present in the greatest quantity.

ALL STAR TIP

- If two flours are listed, the first will be at least 51%.
- If you want 100% whole-wheat bread, no other flour should be listed.
- If it says wheat berries or cracked wheat on the wrapper, you should be able to see them.

- If the wrapper lists the nutrient breakdown, look for bread with 2 to 3 grams of fibre per serving.
- If a bread states it contains "no cholesterol," ignore this claim. Most breads don't contain cholesterol anyway. Cholesterol comes from animal foods.

Bread on the rise

Boosting your fibre intake is easy if you get into the habit of buying whole-grain bread. Two slices (about 50 grams) of whole-grain bread can give you a mighty 3–6 grams of fibre. Since you're aiming for 25–35 grams a day, you can get a significant amount from the bread you eat.

PENNY WISE

Help buns and bread keep their freshness when you're buying them from bulk bins. Store crusty ones in paper bags and soft ones in plastic bags.

ALL STAR TIP

Soft corn or flour tortillas make a great base for tacos, salads or Mexican pizza. All contain less fat than the crispy kind.

fat Budget

Limit muffins that are larger than a cupcake. A large muffin usually contains more than 2 teaspoons of fat.

DID YOU KNOW

Muffin mania began in the 1970s when the news about fibre first came to the fore. Bran, fibre...it all sounded so healthy. In fact, most muffins contain relatively little bran (and some none at all). More to the point, many can be loaded with fat and calories.

Q *What about pancake mixes?*

A For many people it's a weekend tradition—and mixes make it so easy. Pancakes are an OK option; they contain very little fat. But watch the amount that's added at the table. Two tips that work in my house: be more generous with the syrup than the spread. It has half the calories. Switch to a non-hydrogenated, low-fat margarine. It's easier to spread so you use less.

HeartSmart Tip Check your favourite cookbook for a classic pancake recipe, then make some HeartSmart switches:

- Egg whites—2 for each whole egg
- Lower-fat milk instead of whole milk
- Whole-wheat flour instead of white
- Add wheat bran and wheat germ to increase the fibre
- Reduce the oil
- Cook in a nonstick pan

How do I choose bread that contains fibre?

"Wheat flour," "wheat bread," or "cracked wheat" on the wrapper only mean that the bread is made from flour that comes from wheat. It guarantees little more than the term "white flour." Choose "whole wheat" or "stone ground." Oat-bran breads and oat cereals are rich in soluble fibre. The bran in oats is soluble and if eaten in adequate quantities has been shown to help to reduce blood cholesterol.

If a label says a bread contains 100% whole-wheat flour does it mean that 100% of it is whole wheat?

No. Many breads are made with more than one flour. The whole wheat itself may be 100% but there may only be a small amount of it. Check the ingredient list to see what other flours are listed and where the whole wheat is found on the list.

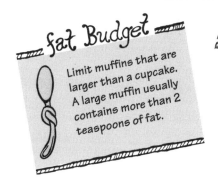

Does dark coloured bread mean that it's high in fibre?

Unfortunately, colour isn't a reliable clue. Bread can be made with refined flour and the dough darkened with molasses, caramel or cocoa. Taking a good look at the label will help.

Banana breads and zucchini loaves sound wonderfully healthy. Are they?

We picture fresh fruits and vegetables when we hear their names. Vitamin rich. Fibre galore. Unfortunately, the rest of the ingredients are often the same as those in regular cake. Very little fruit or vegetable may be used. Try a home-made, lower-fat variety instead.

ALL STAR TIP

- Add wheat germ to up the nutritional value of all-purpose refined flour. Use whole-grain flour whenever possible.
- To make your own self-rising flour, add 1 tablespoon (15 mL) baking powder and 1/4 teaspoon (1 mL) salt to 3 cups (750 mL) flour.

The serious shopper's guide to cereals

Cereal can be the foundation of a fast, nutritious breakfast. Ready-to-eat cereal with lower-fat milk is a good snack for growing youngsters and teens, but it can also be an overload of fat and added sugar. Fortunately, the label tells all. Choose wisely. A good rule of thumb? The shorter the ingredient list the better.

So what's a typical serving size?

A typical serving size is 1 ounce or 1/2 cup (125 mL) for whole grains, 2 cups (500 mL) for puffed and 1/4 cup (50 mL) for granolas. If you eat more than that amount, adjust the values on the label accordingly.

Looking for more fibre?

Choose a cereal that has at least 2 grams of fibre per serving. The fibre will be listed under carbohydrate content. Cereal is a great way to increase your daily fibre intake. A high-fibre cereal has 4 grams of fibre per serving, and you can obtain as much as 9 grams per serving from some all-bran varieties. Granolas may have less fibre than you think. When whole grain is the first ingredient, it's present in the greatest quantity.

Cutting back on fat?

Most cereals are low in fat since they are based on grains, which contain little fat. Ideally they should contain no more than 1 to 3 grams of fat per serving. Granolas may have 5 grams or more, and the fat is often highly saturated coconut or palm oil, or partly saturated hydrogenated vegetable oil. Nuts and seeds add to the fat content. Check the label and look for lower-fat varieties.

Looking for added vitamins and minerals?

Cereal is typically fortified with 10 to 25% of some of the daily vitamins and minerals we require. A great idea, because cereal is the way that many of us start every day. But do you need the "new and improved" cereals that claim to be fortified with 100% of the vitamins and minerals? Not really. Cereal is not all you will be eating during the day. You will get vitamins and minerals from many other food sources. The milk you add will also contain added minerals and vitamins.

Are cereals that contain oats a wild idea?

In fact, they're a good one. Oat bran may reduce blood cholesterol levels. It contains soluble fibre. You have to consume a lot to make a significant difference—about six servings of oats daily, but every bit helps. Try oats in many forms. Old-fashioned rolled oats, quick-cooking rolled oats and instant oats all have similar nutritional value.

Instant oatmeal retains most of the nutrient value of whole and rolled oats, but usually has salt and sugar added to it

Commercial brands of granola and muesli can be high in fat (granola usually more so than muesli). They're often high in tropical oils and include added ingredients such as coconut, nuts and seeds. Read the label and choose the newer low-fat options.

ALL STAR TIP

Try sprinkling fibre on your cereal

- WHEAT BRAN is the outer shell of the wheat kernel. It is the most concentrated form of insoluble fibre there is. Go slowly. Adding too much too fast can affect your body's absorption of calcium and iron, and cause gas and bloating. Allow your body to adapt by increasing your wheat bran intake gradually.
- WHEAT GERM is the embryo of the wheat kernel. It's high in polyunsaturated fat and vitamin E and B vitamins. Store in the fridge so it won't go rancid. Defatted wheat germ (it contains less vitamin E) can be kept in your cupboard.

Pasta...eat oodles of noodles!

Pasta has sat on the side of our dinner plates for long enough. As the fastest growing product in this food group, pasta is not only delicious and versatile, but it's digested slowly so you don't feel the need to snack between meals. Linguini, fettuccini, orzo, penne, rotini, angel hair, rigatoni, pasta shaped like ears, pasta shaped like bows—you can never get bored with pasta.

Convenience? You can't beat it. Twelve minutes in the pot for dry pasta and you can have a bountiful bowl on the table. No wonder we want to find out more.

Pasta may have been the very first convenience food. Three thousand years ago, the Greeks and Romans discovered how to make pastas out of water and ground grain, which they could dry and take with them on long journeys.

All Star Tip

- Pastas called "noodles" contain some egg solids—some cholesterol but not enough to concern yourself about if you rarely choose them.
- Asian noodles are sometimes called imitation noodles because they are not made with egg. They include bean thread noodles, buckwheat noodles (soba), "egg" noodles, rice noodles and wheat noodles.
- Most pasta is made from wheat. If you are allergic to wheat, look for pasta made with other grains.

The instant appeal of instant noodles

I'll admit, oriental instant noodles (e.g., Japanese ramen) are quick, tasty, made in a minute. Precooked and then dried, they are packaged with a packet of seasonings. All you have to do is add boiling water. Yes, they're simple but be careful; they're not that nutritious. These noodles are usually deep-fried in highly saturated fat such as lard or palm oil, and they are high in salt.

fat Budget

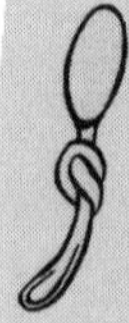

One cup (250 mL) of instant noodles = 3 teaspoons fat.

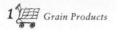

HeartSmart Tip

Choose whole-wheat pasta and double your fibre intake from 2 to 4 grams per cup.

Try "new kinds" of noodles

- High-protein pasta made with soy flour
- Whole-wheat pasta high in fibre and minerals
- No-yolk egg noodles

QA

What are most pastas made from?

The hard spring wheat called durum is unsuitable for breads and cakes but ideal for pasta. The durum wheat is refined and ground into a white flour called semolina. When mixed with water and made into a dough, it can be cut into a vast range of shapes and sizes. Semolina has more protein, vitamins and minerals than ordinary all-purpose flour. It cooks up firm and slightly chewy, or as they say in Italy, *al dente*.

Is fresh pasta a better choice than dried pasta?

Not necessarily. Fresh pasta contains more water, so you get less, kilo for kilo, for your money. Dried pasta can be stored for a long time without any nutrient loss. Cooked or fresh pasta can be frozen for later use.

What gives pasta its different colours and textures?

Often vegetables—beets, carrots or spinach—are used to add colour. Seasoning such as chili peppers or lemon can add another dimension to pasta. Whole-wheat pastas have a different texture and taste (they need longer cooking) but they do contain more fibre, vitamins and minerals and have a slightly higher protein content.

How can I find a sauce that's low in fat?

Many labels don't supply nutrition information, so your best bet is to read the ingredient list and think about your fat budget if cream, cheese, meats or fats are listed near the top.

What are good ways to boost your pasta sauces?

Not by adding cream, butter or cheese—which means limit that Fettuccini Alfredo! Use a tomato sauce as a base, and add tuna or scallops, or make a luscious and authentically Italian primavera sauce with fresh vegetables steamed briefly and a touch of white wine. Delicious.

fun food...fast

Momma Ramona's fresh tomato sauce

This is a cinch to make and it explodes with flavour. Serves four.

2 tsp (10 mL) olive oil—or use stock
2 cloves garlic, finely chopped
1 1/2 lb (750 g) chopped firm roma tomatoes or a 28 oz (796 g) can tomatoes
big pinch basil, parsley, oregano, rosemary
salt and pepper to taste
1 tbsp (15 mL) parmesan cheese

Heat oil in nonstick frying pan. Sauté garlic until lightly browned. Add tomatoes and cook until tomatoes release some juice. Break tomatoes up with a wooden spoon. Stir in herbs (use at least double for fresh herbs) and cook for about 5 minutes, until sauce reduces. Season to taste. Serve immediately over cooked pasta. One tablespoon of grated parmesan cheese provides less than 1/2 tsp fat and just 25 calories. Or try the new lower-fat parmesan cheese. Enjoy!

Cooking rice and other grains

Rice is *really* nice nutritionally. When we were growing up, most of us viewed rice as an extra—the little white mound on the side of the plate. Yet half the world eats rice as its staple food. Chinese tradition has it that a person who has not eaten rice has not fully eaten.

Rice is easy to cook. Measure it first, allowing about 1/3 cup (75 mL) per person. Rinse thoroughly until water runs clear. Place in a pot and add twice the amount of water or add flavour by using broth or juice instead of water. Bring to a boil, stir well, cover and reduce heat. Simmer for 20 minutes. Fluff rice with a fork before serving so that the steam can escape and the grains don't stick together.

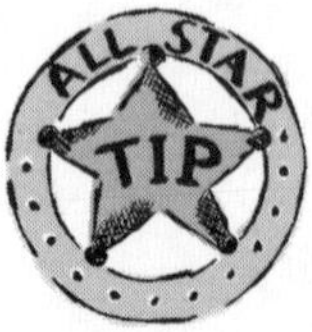

If you cannot serve rice immediately, cover with a tea towel and place the lid back on—this will prevent rice turning gummy.

fun food...fast

Quick and nippy rice recipes

Rice Pilaf

Sauté 1 chopped onion in 1 tbsp (15 mL) of hot stock. Add 1 cup (250 mL) rice and cook two minutes until rice becomes opaque. Add 2 cups (500mL) boiling stock. Cover and cook until liquid is absorbed. Season with cinnamon and ginger. Toss with a scant handful of chopped nuts or dried fruit.

Vegetable Paella

Sauté 1 chopped onion, a chopped garlic clove and 1 cup (250 mL) uncooked rice in 2 tbsp (25 mL) hot stock until onions are transparent and rice lightly browned. Add 1 1/2 cups (375 mL) boiling stock, 1 cup (250 mL) stewed tomatoes with juice, and a pinch of paprika, cayenne pepper and crushed saffron. Bring to boil, reduce heat and simmer 10 minutes. Add a chopped-up pepper, 1/2 cup (125 mL) each of frozen peas and corn niblets. Cover and simmer again for 10 minutes until liquid is absorbed and rice is tender.

Green Rice

Add freshly chopped parsley or cilantro to cooked rice. Experiment with other herbs.

Main Meal Rice

Simply mix in cut-up cooked vegetables, lean meat or chicken. A great way to stretch leftovers.

White rice, brown rice. Short grain, long grain. Red rice, wild rice. What a fabulous way to add variety to the foods we eat.

White rice makes up nearly 99% of the rice we eat. Too bad. Even in Asia, nearly all the rice eaten is polished, which strips it of fibre, protein, vitamins and minerals.

DID YOU KNOW?

Different shapes of rice give different results when you cook them. The shorter the grain, the stickier the rice. Long grains are ideal for casseroles and stuffing.

What's the scoop on brown rice?

Choose good and chewy brown or whole-grain rice and you're getting the whole unpolished rice grain. Only the husk and a little of the bran is removed. Though it takes a bit longer to cook than white rice, it contains more fibre and minerals. Unlike other rice, it's also a source of vitamin E.

HeartSmart Tip

How much fibre in a cup of rice?

1 cup	*Fibre*
White rice	1 g
Brown rice	3 g
Wild rice	4 g

Choose brown rice over white rice and increase your fibre intake from 1 gram to 3 grams per cup.

What's the word on parboiled or converted rice?

The word is yes! This rice goes through a special steam-pressure process which pushes some of its nutrients into the starchy centre of each grain so that vitamins are not lost when the rice is milled. Unfortunately it is lower in fibre than brown rice. The word "parboiled" might lead you to think that this kind of rice cooks quickly. In fact, it takes just as long to cook as ordinary rice.

Any thoughts on precooked or instant rice?

These are the most highly processed and expensive rices. Even when enriched, they offer the least nourishment.

fat Budget

If you use a packaged rice mix, you don't need to add fat even though the box says to. The rice tastes fine without it—and that would help your fat budget. It is also just as simple to make your own seasoned rice from scratch using your favourite herbs.

Grains galore

It's time to spread the word. The best kept secret around is all the deliciously different grains you'll find in your supermarket. Popular staples of Middle Eastern and Mediterranean cuisine, most of them cook in a flash—often faster than rice or pasta.

Amaranth An ancient Aztec grain. The only grain that supplies a good amount of calcium. Good source of iron too. Each kernel is as tiny as a poppy seed. Most appetizing when added to another grain. Cook in broth or juice and combine with stir-fries.

Barley Delicious in soups (see recipe on page 122), stews, casseroles, and as a cereal. Whole (Scotch) barley is more nutritious than the polished (pearl) barley and takes longer to cook.

Buckwheat This is actually a seed. Whole, it's called groats. Roasted and ground, it's known as kasha. Before cooking, add beaten egg to coat the grains—this will prevent the grains from sticking together. To cut the added fat, use beaten egg whites.

Quinoa Pronounced "keen-wa," this is a light, non-sticky grain with a delicate flavour. Substitute for rice or use as a base for salads. It is called the mother grain because it has more complete protein than any other grain and is high in vitamins and minerals. Not as expensive as it may seem because it increases 3 to 4 times during cooking. It's cooked when grains are translucent and turn into spirals.

Cornmeal Ground corn kernels. Make Italian polenta by bringing 3 cups of lightly salted water or stock to a boil, then slowly pour in 1 cup of cornmeal (to prevent lumps, add a little water to the cornmeal first, blend and then add). Stir constantly until mixture starts to come away from the sides of the pan. Can be pressed in pan, cut into squares and broiled.

Wheat *Wheat berries*—the whole-wheat kernels are high in nutrition. Enjoy as a cereal or add to breads and muffins. Keep in the fridge because the whole grain contains natural oils which can turn rancid.

Bulgur—or cracked wheat, often called the rice of the Middle East. Can be served in many innovative ways—as a main event, side dish or cold salad.

Couscous—a North African specialty, is made from semolina and is actually a form of pasta. Add to boiling water, turn heat off and leave to cook.

Quick guide to cooking grains (check package for instructions)

GRAINS (1 CUP)	WATER	TIME (MINUTES)
Amaranth	1 cup (250 mL)	30
Barley		
Scotch (whole)	4 cups (1 L)	100
Pearl (polished)	3 cups (750 mL)	55
Buckwheat		
Groats (whole)	2 cups (500 mL)	15
Kasha (roasted, hulled)	5 cups (1.25 mL)	12
Millet	3 cups (750 mL)	30
Oats		
Whole	2 cups (500 mL)	60
Rolled	2 cups (500 mL)	10
Quinoa	2 cups (500 mL)	15
Rice		
Long grain	2 cups (500 mL)	20
Short grain	2 cups (500 mL)	20
White basmati	1 1/2 cups (375 mL)	15
Wild rice	4 cups (1 L)	50
Wheat		
Wheat berries	3 cups (750 mL)	60
Bulgur	2 cups (500 mL)	15
Couscous	2 cups (500 mL)	15

fun food...fast

Great grain boosters

- To boost flavour, cook grains in broth or diluted orange or tomato juice.
- For an Asian twist, season with soy sauce, ground sesame seeds and grated ginger. Or try curry powder with chopped cilantro, peppers, green onion and orange slices. For a Mediterranean flavour add oregano, basil, marjoram and chopped parsley.
- For a tasty hot meal or side dish, toss cooked grains with cooked vegetables (e.g., carrots, celery, mushrooms), fresh herbs and your favourite low-fat dressing.
- For delicious cold salads, add cold cooked grains to tuna, chopped vegetables (e.g., peas, mushrooms, peppers, green onions) and toss with a vinaigrette dressing or lemon juice and a dash of olive oil.
- For tasty thickened soups, add grains to stock pot.
- To get used to the nutty flavour of many of these grains, combine them with milder grains, e.g., add brown rice to kasha (roasted buckwheat).

Cookies? Pastries?

OK, the truth. No way can you justify cookies and pastries from a nutritional standpoint—they're usually loaded with fat and calories. But who eats them for nutrition anyway? In fact, statistics reveal that each of us eats about 5 kilograms of cookies a year! Balance your cookie craving by keeping a close eye on the other fats you eat that day. That way you'll still have your fat budget under control.

Cookies contain flour, fat and sugar. Your best bets are those that are high in whole-wheat flour and low in fat and calories.

Some cookie facts

No matter what fat is used, the less the better.

Fat-free cookies may still be loaded with sugar. Read the label, and check the calories per serving.

ALL STAR TIP

- A cookie that is "calorie reduced" means that it has fewer calories than the original product—but it doesn't necessarily mean that it's low in calories. Once again, let the label be your guide and compare with other choices.
- "Whole-grain" on granola bars means they may contain a small quantity of oats, but the amount may be insignificant relative to the added fat and calories.

DID YOU KNOW

Made with oats, nuts and seeds, granola bars are high in protein and fibre. They may seem to be a wise choice but in fact they are usually high in fat and calories too—often boosted by other ingredients such as miniature marshmallows, or chocolate or caramel chips. Check the label to learn the fat and calories in a serving size. Enjoy them if you want, but keep your fat budget in mind—and choose the new products lower in fat and calories.

Some of the wisest choices in the cookie aisle are some of the oldest ones. Gingersnaps and graham crackers are both low in fat. So are fruit bars, wafers and animal crackers. The good news . . . manufacturers know we can't resist the cookie jar so they're hard at work inventing cookies that are lower in fat and calories. Keep your eyes open.

Putting the crunch on crackers

Crackers can be a wise choice if you're watching your calorie, fat and fibre intake. But how do you know which to pick?

- Look for as little fat and salt as possible.
- Choose crackers made from whole-grain flour whenever you can.
- Read the ingredients and make sure that whole-wheat flour is top of the list.

Big crackers, small crackers, ones you can eat by the handful, ones that take several bites—no wonder a serving size of crackers is anybody's guess. Only you know how many you eat at a time. Try to get the most crackers you can for the fewest calories.

Cracker countdown

These are all good choices:

- Flatbreads and crispbreads
- Water crackers
- Rice cakes
- Melba toasts
- Matzos

ALL STAR TIP

If a cracker is greasy to the touch or leaves a greasy mark on paper, it's high in fat.

Grains at a glance

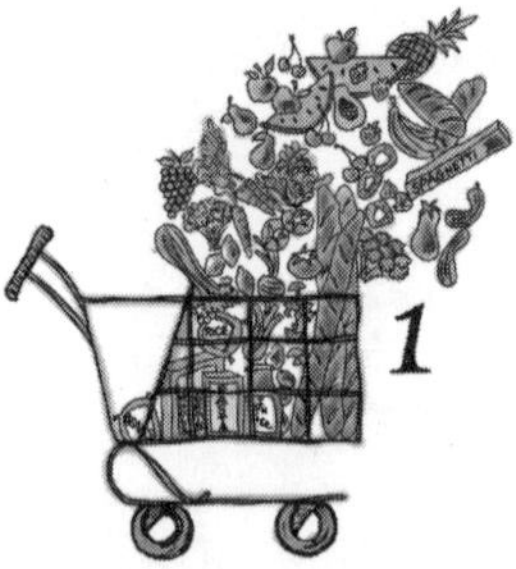

1. Look for whole-grain products.
2. Choose cereals with at least 2 grams fibre per serving.
3. Experiment with varieties of grains.

VEGETABLES & FRUIT

Feel free to fill the big #1 part of your cart, loading it up with veggies and fruit

Hope you left lots of space in the large #1 part of your shopping cart, because here's where HeartSmart shoppers can really go crazy. Run riot! Fill your cart to the top. Along with grain products, vegetables and fruit should form the bulk of your diet.

We all grew up being told to eat our vegetables and somewhere along the line, we got the idea that they weren't delicious. A crispy green salad? Sweet little peas just out of the pod? A snappy handful of carrot sticks? Tiny new potatoes? *Not delicious?!!*

Vegetables can be b-o-o-oring if you serve the same ones day after day, especially at the end of the season. So try some new faces. From blue potatoes to yellow tomatoes, your supermarket is brimming with different varieties. Try scarlet kale or chopped red cabbage to jazz up a plain green salad. Add colour to mashed potatoes with a handful of parsley—vibrant green and available year round. Zip up a fish dish with jalapeno peppers. Even a little makes a huge difference.

And think about fruit. Bite into a juicy sun-warmed peach. Chill out with cold cubes of honeydew on a hot summer day. Picture the sharp yellows and greens of lemons and limes piled in a wicker basket. Wander the world of tropical fruit. Try chunks of papaya on your breakfast cereal (and use the seeds in salad dressing, see page 61). Serve yellow-orange slices of gorgeous mango for dessert. Snack on a bowl of lychees when they're in season.

No wonder supermarkets display their produce with pride. In fact, it's the only section so beautiful that it often gets to look at itself in a mirror. We often judge where we shop by how fresh and attractive its produce looks. Fruits and vegetables are loaded with nutrients. Antioxidants, phytochemicals, complex carbohydrates, fibre—they're full of the substances that we can feel free to eat in abundance. And oh, so low in fat.

Want some proof? Over one hundred studies now confirm that plant foods play a special role in the prevention of heart disease, obesity and cancer.

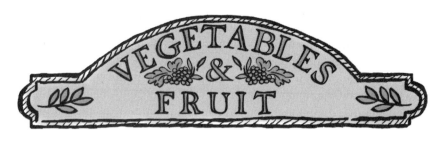

Take five! And more if you can

Canada's Food Guide to Healthy Eating recommends 5 to 10 servings a day from the produce section. If that sounds like a lot, relax, it isn't.

One serving means:

1 medium fruit or vegetable	1/2 cup (125 mL) fruit juice
1/2 cup (125 mL) cooked vegetables	1 cup salad

ALL STAR TIP

1 serving fruit or vegetable = the size of a tennis ball

Here's how 10 servings might work for you and your family on a typical day.

Breakfast: a small glass of orange juice or half a grapefruit
Mid-morning: an apple
Lunch: minestrone soup, or a large salad, lettuce and tomato in your sandwich
Supper: soup or salad plus one or two cups of vegetables, fresh grapes or a half cantaloupe for dessert
Snack: frozen berries or a banana

Fat budgeting with vegetables and fruits

Most vegetables and fruits are low in fat. That's why it's so easy to load up the #1 part of your cart. Choose a variety to get a range of important nutrients.

Check the fat budget list and decide how you want to spend your fat budget.

Fat Budget

Vegetables and fruits:

0 tsp. fat	most vegetables and fruits fruit and vegetable juices

1 tsp. fat	2 tbsp (25 mL) shredded coconut 7 olives
2 tsp. fat	1/2 cup (125 mL) hash browns 10 french fries
3 tsp. fat	1/2 medium avocado

1 teaspoon fat = approximately 5 grams of fat.
These numbers are averages.

To find out what nutrients vegetables and fruit offer and where they fit in the total nutrition picture, see Appendix, page 124.

fat Budget

- What about fruit pies? Too high in fat to be considered a fruit serving. Sorry.
- Go slow with french fries. Made from potatoes, yes, but the added fat can burden your fat budget.
- The fat in olives and avocadoes is mostly monounsaturated — a wise way to spend your fat budget.

ALL STAR TIP

"A palette for your palate" is the ideal way to balance your fruit and vegetables. Fill your cart with as many different colours as you can. Green lettuce, broccoli, peas, green beans and zucchini. Yellow squash, grapefruit and bananas. Red sweet peppers, tomatoes and apples. Orange squash and apricots. A wide spectrum of colours means you're getting the full spectrum of nutrients and phytochemicals that fruit and vegetables offer. A bonus—on a plate, all those hues look extra appealing.

Extra! Extra! Read all about them

Fruits and vegetables come in their own gorgeous packaging but if they were sold like other products, imagine what it might say on their labels:

- *High in Fibre!*
- *No Cholesterol!*
- *Low Fat!*
- *With Phytochemicals and Antioxidants!*

What a bonanza. Fruit and vegetables are loaded with nutrients and low in calories. Nice to know if you want to stay healthy and manage your weight.

Eating a diet that contains a healthy amount of fibre may lessen your risk of developing heart disease, constipation, cancer of the colon, rectal cancer and breast cancer, obesity and diverticulosis.

An apple a day? Yes!

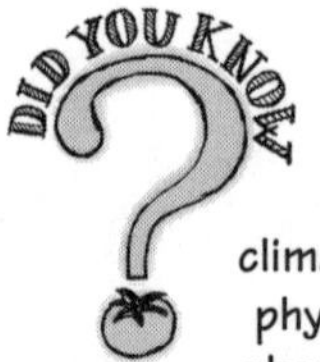

Phytochemicals (fight-o-chemicals) are naturally present in plants. We know that these chemicals protect the plant. They fight the stresses of harsh climate and infections—but we do not yet know how these phytochemicals work in human beings. The research showing their possible benefits is relatively new. Scientists are still trying to unlock the secrets of these potentially exciting nutrients. That's why it's a good idea to add more fruit and vegetables to your diet rather than popping supplements which don't necessarily provide the full spectrum.

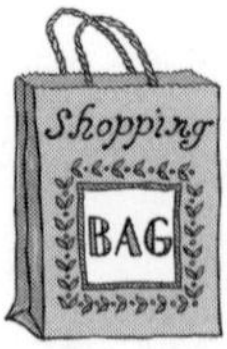

You'll find phytochemicals in:

- Cruciferous vegetables such as broccoli, cauliflower and cabbage
- Legumes, especially soy products
- Flax seed
- Carrots, parsley, parsnips, turnips, citrus fruits
- Garlic, onions, chives

Eat as many different kinds as you can.

Arm yourself with fruit and vegetables

A rusting iron pipe and a cut apple that turns brown might not seem to have much in common. In fact, both are examples of what oxygen does in the wrong place at the wrong time—and something similar can cause damage in our bodies.

The good news? Recent research suggests that three vitamins, A (beta carotene), C and E, may come to the rescue. They are called antioxidants. Fruit and vegetables are loaded with A (in the form of beta carotene) and C.

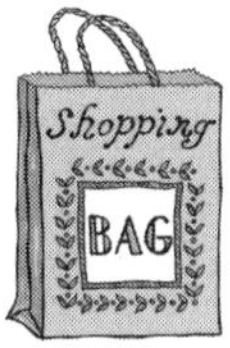

You'll find beta carotene in:

- Dark green leafy vegetables such as collard greens, spinach, mustard greens, kale, broccoli and Swiss chard
- Yellow and orange vegetables such as carrots, squash, pumpkins and sweet potatoes
- Yellow and orange fruits such as melons, apricots, mangoes, papaya and peaches

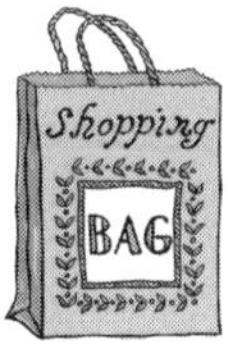

You'll find vitamin C in:

- Vegetables: peppers, cauliflower, broccoli, brussels sprouts, sweet potatoes and snow peas
- Fruits: citrus fruits, strawberries, papaya, melon and kiwis
- Juice from these fruits or juice enriched with vitamin C

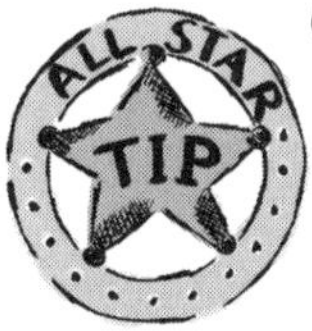

Choose deep orange or dark green vegetables and fruits at least every other day to help you get enough antioxidants.

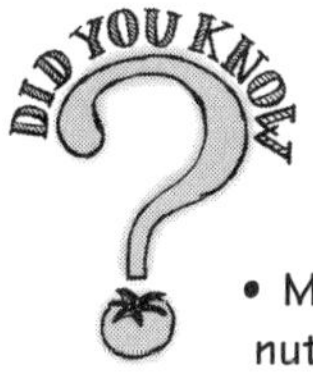

- Don't be fooled by beta carotene look-alikes. Sweet corn and beets may be the right colour but their colour doesn't come from beta carotene. Still good choices, but not for beta carotene.
- Many foods high in vitamin E are also high in fat—vegetable oils, nuts and seeds, margarine, wheat germ.

QA

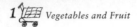

How about frozen fruit?

Feel free to buy it. Picked and chilled at its prime, frozen fruit has the same nutrients as fresh. The trip from orchard to freezer often takes only a few hours. Frozen fruits are processed without cooking and so there is little if any nutrient loss. Give those frozen raspberries a shake before they go in your cart. A rattling sound means they haven't thawed, then refrozen. And remember to check the label—sometimes sugar is added, which boosts the calories.

What about canned fruit and vegetables?

An easy, penny-wise way to add colour to your plate, canned fruits and veggies are super convenient—and they offer variety year round. Canned products today retain much of their vitamins and minerals, though water-soluble vitamins run the risk of being destroyed by the high temperatures called for in the canning process.

Get the most out of your canned vegetables and fruit

ALL STAR TIP

- Minerals such as calcium or iron may have leached into the canning liquid. You can add it to soups or use it instead of water when you put the rice pot on, but remember canned vegetables are often heavily salted. Look for "low salt" on the label.
- Canned fruits may be packed in syrup which doubles the calorie content. Choose water-packed or juice-packed varieties instead.

Should I add dried fruit to my shopping list?

Raisins, dried apricots, dried apples—all those lusciously sweet dried fruits are delicious, and a good idea added to cereals or tossed in salads. Not only that, they're packed with fruity nutrients. Minerals like iron, copper and potassium. Vitamins too (though vitamin C is often lost.) That's the good news. Everything else is concentrated too including the calories. Eat in small amounts. If you are allergic to sulfites, avoid dried fruits such as raisins, prunes and peaches which may have sulfites added to prevent browning. Look for sulfite-free varieties.

Peeled, cut and bagged veggies are so convenient. Am I losing out on nutrients?

When you're stuck for time, this is a wonderful way to save minutes in the kitchen without much loss in nutrients. The downside? Prepackaged veggies do cost a bit more. Make sure that you buy fresh produce, refrigerate it, and eat by the "best before" date.

How can I protect my family from pesticide residues in fruit and vegetables?

- Buy local produce.
- Eat what is in season.
- Choose a variety to minimize your exposure to any one pesticide.
- Unless you're going to peel them, scrub all fruit and vegetables and rinse thoroughly.
- Peel oranges and grapefruit with a knife; do not bite into peel.
- Throw away the outer leaves of leafy vegetables such as lettuce and cabbage and the leaves at the top of vegetables such as celery and cauliflower.
- Peel waxed fruit and vegetables when possible. While safe in themselves, waxes seal in fungicide or pesticide residues.

Organic foods

In Canada, foods that say "organically grown" or "certified organic" must meet standards set by government and local independent agencies. Buying organic produce is a vote for a certain kind of agriculture that replenishes the soil, and protects the water supply and the people who work in the fields. Many people believe that organic foods offer extra nutrition. To be honest, we don't know. The nutrient content of a food is determined more by its genes, the climate, when it was picked and how it was shipped and stored than by the type of fertilizer used or soil in which it was grown.

Organic foods often cost more, and produce may not look as perfect as the kind you find in your supermarket. Those who do buy organic say that the flavour is better. It's a personal choice—and an environmentally friendly decision.

Fresh fruit and vegetables contain essential nutrients that may actually help your body resist disease, prevent cancer and resist the ravages of chemical pollution. Organic or not, eat plenty of fruit and vegetables.

KIDSTUFF

Spinach? Yuck!

You can't force kids to eat foods they don't like, but you can persuade them—subtly. If they're old enough, suggest that they help you prepare the vegetables for supper. (Even little ones can have fun tearing up lettuce leaves for a family salad.) When you've actually peeled the carrots yourself, it's tough to say no when they show up on your plate. Speaking of carrots, kids usually prefer vegetables that are brightly coloured and crunchy. Carrots, of course, but also red pepper strips, snow peas, broccoli flowers, new green beans, the list goes on. Kids often prefer their vegetables raw—less work for you! Served up on a platter with a creamy low-fat dip, they're much more fun.

Tell your kids they're going skinny-dipping! Just mix equal parts of low-fat mayonnaise and low-fat yogurt, and season to taste with ketchup or powdered soup mix.

DID YOU KNOW

- Cruciferous vegetables are said to help in protecting against certain forms of cancer. Cruciferous comes from the word "cross." These vegetables have a cross-shaped flower. They include cabbage, broccoli, brussels sprouts, cauliflower, kohlrabi (that vegetable that looks like a sputnik), kale and turnips.

- Fruit gets sweeter with age. Vegetables get starchy. As fruit matures, its starch is converted into sugar. As vegetables mature, the sugar turns into starch, and they become drier and mealier.

ALL STAR TIP

Here's a tip to help fruit ripen faster. Don't put fruit out in the sun because heat and light can cause nutrient loss. Instead, punch some holes in a brown paper bag, put the fruit inside and leave it in a cool place. Adding an apple to the bag also speeds up the ripening process. Apples give off ethylene, a natural gas that causes fruit to ripen. In fact, this gas is often used to ripen fruit on its way from orchard to table. It isn't harmful. Because of this ripening action, apples need to be kept away from fruit that is already at its peak. Keeping fruit in the fridge will slow the ripening process.

Veg out whenever you can

Fresh vegetables are a wonderfully easy way to boost your fibre and vitamin intake. And you can't beat them for value. Buy vegetables in season when they're at their peak. That way, you'll get maximum flavour. And use them fresh.

The closer a vegetable is grown to your home, the better it usually tastes. After all, you know how you feel after three or four days on the road! Preparing salad greens night after night can be a chore. Instead, why not do the basics as soon as you unpack your shopping? Wash lettuce and other greens. Store them in plastic bags (with a paper towel added to absorb any moisture). Then tear into pieces when you need them. What you might lose in vitamin C you will save in time. Your choice.

Is it fresh? How to give veggies the eye!

Artichokes Look for those with tightly closed leaves and no bruises. Squeeze them. Fresh artichokes squeak.

Asparagus Bright green stalks with closed pointed tips are at their peak. Cold water or refrigeration keeps them fresh in the supermarket. You do the same.

Avocado Flawless skin is what you want. If hard, leave to ripen on the counter. If soft, store in the fridge. Remember, an avocado has 3 teaspoons of monounsaturated fat.

Beans Buy them loose if you can and pick out those with bright colour and velvety feel. If they're full of beans, forget 'em. They'll be old and tough.

Beets Full and firm is what you're looking for. Try to buy them with the greens attached. Steam and serve those separately for a nutritional jumpstart.

Bok Choy Also called Chinese mustard cabbage. Stalks should be firm and white, topped with deep green, veined leaves. Cooking cuts the sharp tang of the leaves and sweetens the stalks.

Broccoli Stalks should look tender and crisp and should snap easily. Florets should be green—the darker the better. Yellow means they're past it. Cook fast to cut down on cooking smells. Keep the beta-carotene-rich leaves for your soup pot.

Brussels sprouts Deeply coloured, tightly packed leaves mean freshness. Any little holes? A worm got there first.

Cabbage Green or red, choose firm and heavy heads with tightly closed leaves. As with brussels sprouts, watch for evidence of worms.

Carrots Leave limp, pale carrots in the bin. Chop off any tops before you put them away so they can't draw moisture away from the carrots.

Cauliflower White, firm, clean looking florets and bright green leaves mean freshness.

Celery Choose firm, tightly closed bunches with light green leaves. Dark green celery is often stringy.

Corn Pull back the husk and check for plump, firm, tightly packed kernels.

Cucumber Look for bright green colour and firmness. Watch for shrivelled ends.

Eggplant The skin should be as smooth as dark purple satin. Firm, heavy eggplants are your best choice. Leave behind any with soft spots or bruises. A small "navel" at the bottom means fewer seeds inside.

Garlic Heads should be firm and heavy with no green sprouts or soft spots.

Greens For cooking greens like kale, chard and mustard greens, pick the freshest looking leaves you can find and as vividly coloured as possible. Remove the outside leaves.

For salad greens, rinse and dry them well and store wrapped in a tea towel in your vegetable crisper until needed. Dry greens need less dressing.

Mushrooms	Look for tightly closed caps with no soft or bruised areas. Store in a paper bag. Plastic will make them mushy.
Onions	The firmer, the better. Soft spots or green sprouts mean an onion is past its prime.
Peppers	Pick the firmest peppers you can find in the darkest colours. The walls should feel thick.
Potatoes	Not a good buy if the skin is shrivelled, soft, green, or sprouting. Store in a brown paper bag or dark cupboard at room temperature, not in the fridge where their starch will turn to sugar and alter the taste. Cut away any green areas before cooking but eat the skin whenever possible.
Squash (summer)	Thin-skinned and tender, zucchini and baby squash taste sweetest when they're small or medium sized. Look for plump, firm, heavy squash with a bright, uniform colour.
Spinach	Look for small leaves, thin stems and a bright green colour. Should smell sweet, not musty.
Squash (winter)	Rich in beta carotene (vitamin A), acorn, butternut, spaghetti and pumpkin are just a few of this gloriously colourful family. Look for deep colour and smooth rinds free of cracks. Weigh them in your hand—they should feel heavy. Stored in a cool, dark place, winter squash will last for several weeks.
Sui Choy	You may know this as Chinese cabbage or Napa cabbage. Either way, it should be compact and barrel shaped with white, crunchy stalks and crinkly, pale green leaves.
Sweet potatoes	Smooth skin with no wrinkles is what you want. Check that the ends aren't discoloured. Root vegetables are sweeter when smaller.
Tomatoes	Choose them one by one so you can look for firm, plump tomatoes that aren't overripe or blemished. Keep them out on the counter, not in the refrigerator.
Turnips	Small means sweet. Firm and smooth skinned means the best flavour.

ALL STAR TIP

- Double your fibre intake by eating potatoes with the skin on.
- Instead of stir-frying vegetables in oil, try sautéing them in a little stock or low-fat salad dressing.

PENNY WISE

Seven ways to get the most nutrients for your money

1. Prepare fruits and vegetables just before you cook them.
2. Cook vegetables with the skin on.
3. Steam, roast or microwave produce.
4. Cook produce as briefly as possible.
5. Cook large chunks rather than small pieces.
6. Cover and refrigerate juices after opening.
7. Eat raw fruits and vegetables whenever you can.

fun food...fast

Veggie power

Colourful Coleslaw

Mix together thinly sliced red and green cabbage, raisins, chopped apple and a few chopped walnuts. Toss with a mixture of equal parts low-fat mayonnaise and low-fat yogurt.

Sweet Carrots

Steam carrots until tender-crisp. Toss with orange juice and honey and cook until they have a glazed look. Another time, try a mixture of orange marmalade with lemon juice and a dab of margarine. It explodes with flavour.

Nutty Cauliflower

Sauté florets in broth or water and toss with parsley and sliced toasted almonds.

Perfect Corn

Add sugar to the cooking water to enhance the sweetness. Salt toughens the kernels.

Eggplant Secrets Cracked Open

Eggplants absorb oil like a sponge. Reduce the fat you need by broiling or grilling instead of sautéing them. Cut lengthwise into thick slices—there's no need to peel them—prick with a fork and brush with a mixture of oil, chopped garlic and herbs. Turn the slices as they brown.

Need skinless eggplant? Leave whole, or halve the eggplant lengthwise, prick it all over with a fork, place cut side down and broil until skin is blistered and blackened. Place in a paper bag for a few minutes and the skin will peel off easily.

Great English Cucumbers

Just grate them into a bowl, squeeze to remove moisture and add low-fat yogurt, dill, minced garlic and salt to taste.

Homemade Sun-dried Tomatoes

Place sliced tomatoes in a single layer on a cookie sheet. Bake at 400°F (200°C) for about eight minutes until lightly browned and crisp. Store in a jar in the fridge. A wonderful addition to pasta sauces (and only you have to know they weren't dried in the sun).

Oven-roasted Vegetables

Cut eggplant, peppers, mushrooms, butternut squash or zucchini into one inch (2.5 cm) cubes and toss with a mixture of olive oil, garlic and herbs—try balsamic vinegar too. Place skin side up on a baking sheet and roast at 400°F (200°C) until browned, 15 to 30 minutes. Shake the pan a few times as the vegetables cook to prevent sticking. The result? Vegetables with intense flavour, crisp skin and tender flesh.

Use as a salad on crisp lettuce, toss them with pasta or spread on a pizza crust with salsa, low-fat cheese and a sprinkle of parmesan.

Ratatouille

A wonderfully tasty dish originating in France. Sauté large chunks of unpeeled eggplant, tomato, onion, red or green peppers, zucchini and some chopped garlic in a little olive oil. Season with basil, thyme and oregano. Cover and let simmer in its juices for 30 minutes. Make lots. Ratatouille is terrific hot or cold. It can be whizzed in the blender for a fast homemade soup—and it freezes beautifully.

Quick Tomato Salad

Mix chopped tomato, chopped onion and cubed low-fat mozzarella. Drizzle with red wine vinegar and vegetable oil. How's that for simple?

Low-fat French "Fries"

Cut large potatoes into wedges and brush lightly with oil. Sprinkle with basil or paprika. Layer on baking sheet sprayed with nonstick cooking spray or lined with parchment paper. Bake at 450°F (230°C) for 40 minutes. Turn as required.

Great Broiled Potatoes

Cut potatoes in quarters, leaving skins on for increased nutritional value. Microwave for a few minutes until almost cooked. Toss in low-fat Italian dressing. Broil for 2-3 minutes. Turn and broil again. Drizzle with more dressing and serve. Yum!

KIDSTUFF

Ant Logs

Kids love these as a snack! Fill celery stalks with peanut butter and sprinkle with raisins.

Quick! Name the vegetable most North American kids eat most.

The answer? Potatoes. Made into french fries.

Too bad, because then they are loaded in fat. One large potato weighs in at only 180 calories. Turn that potato into french fries and its calorie count rockets to over 600. Check above for low-fat "fries" that kids will love.

fat Budget

Cutting down on french fries saves you 1 tsp fat for 5 regular fries. A bonanza for your fat budget!

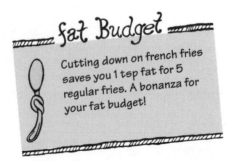

PENNY WISE

Cooking Tips

The longer you boil vegetables, the more vitamins you lose. Steam or microwave vegetables whenever you can and save the water for adding to soups and stocks.

Storage Tips

- Keep most fruit in the fridge to stop the process of ripening.
- Refrigerate green leafy vegetables in vegetable crisper or in moisture-proof bags with a paper towel added.
- Potatoes, carrots, sweet potatoes and other root vegetables keep best in a cool and moist place to prevent withering.
- Quick, before they go bad, freeze leftover raw vegetables for use in soups and stocks.
- Don't let root vegetables wither away. Buy carrots, parsnips, beets, turnips and other cold-weather favourites without their tops, or cut away the greens when you get home. The green leaves look pretty but they suck nutrients and moisture from the roots—the part you want to eat. Save beet greens to steam, or to chop and add to soups or pastas.

fun food...fast

Five ways to give potatoes a-peel

We know that the usual blobs of butter or sour cream aren't a good idea. No problem. Here are five healthy ways to dress up a potato.

- Top baked potatoes with low-fat yogurt seasoned with flavoured vinegar, parsley, green onions.
- Sprinkle new potatoes with chopped green onions, chives, fresh dill or rosemary.
- Grind some black pepper and add a few drops of sesame oil for an intriguing Asian twist, or add just a few drops of lower salt soy sauce.
- Try a dab of low-fat margarine mixed with lemon juice or Dijon mustard.
- Blend soup stock or wine into mashed potatoes, plus puréed cooked vegetables. Try broccoli, asparagus and zucchini for starters.

Put the squeeze on fresh fruit

Buying fruits loose rather than bagged lets you choose each one individually.

Apples	If you can dent it with your finger, don't buy it.
Bananas	They ripen with time, so buy as you need them—green for later in the week, ripe for snacking while you unpack.
Berries	If the box is damp or stained, look for another one. It means that the bottom layers of fruit are decaying. Buy uncrushed berries with no mould. Buy strawberries loose if you can and choose each one individually.
Cherries	Buy them ripe and avoid any sticky ones. They will damage the others.
Grapefruit	Firm and springy is what you're looking for. Weigh one against another in your hands. Thin-skinned ones that feel heavy for their size are juicier.
Grapes	If they look plump and good enough to eat, they are. Stems should be green and supple.
Kiwi	Press them gently. If they yield, they're ripe.
Lemons and Limes	Choose firm, plump ones that are heavy for their size, rich in colour and have a slightly glossy skin.
Mangoes	Choose firm and unblemished fruit that smells sweet and yields to gentle pressure. Note: wash your hands after touching them—mangoes contain a chemical that you may be sensitive to.
Melons: Honeydew and Cantaloupe	Look for dull, velvety skin. Then check the top. A sunken, smooth scar means they were picked ripe. The bottom should yield slightly to pressure. Smell the aroma. You can buy melons underripe too and let them ripen at room temperature.
Nectarines	Pick plump nectarines that are slightly soft along the seam. Hard, green nectarines may not ripen.

Oranges Choose ones that are firm, heavy and free from spots and wrinkles

Papayas Look for those that are mostly yellow and have a pleasant smell. Press them gently. They should give slightly, but shouldn't feel soft.

Peaches A distinct peachy aroma and slightly soft fruit is what you're looking for. Buy peaches as you want to eat them, ripe or nearly ripe. Once off the tree, they won't ripen any more.

Pears Pick firm, unbruised pears that yield to pressure. Colour doesn't matter. You can even buy them green and let them ripen at room temperature.

Pineapples Squeeze them gently with your fingertips. They should give a little.

Plums Think plums, think plump and slightly soft with perfect skins. Buy them ripe.

Rhubarb Choose firm, crisp stalks and chop off the leaves.

Watermelon At its best when the surface is smooth with a dullish sheen and the underside is a creamy yellow. Its ends should yield slightly when you press them. The final test? Slap it. A dull, flat sound means an underripe watermelon. A hollow noise tells you it's past its best.

Kiwi fruits and apples produce ethylene gas which will cause the fruit around them to ripen faster. Keep them separate—unless you want this effect.

PENNY WISE

If pineapples are all the same price but different sizes, pick the biggest one. Their skin is all the same thickness so you'll get more fruit for your money.

fun food...fast

Simple sunny fresh fruit

Granny Smith's Best Baked Apples

This homey dessert will fill your kitchen with the wonderful aroma of melted cinnamon and brown sugar. The best apple variety to use is Granny Smith.

Core the apple, fill with a mixture of cinnamon, a small amount of sugar and raisins. Place in a baking dish, add a little water, cover and bake at 350°F (180°C) for 30 minutes. Remove cover and bake for 30 minutes longer.

Note: to help apples keep their shape while cooking, run a knife around the middle of each one so that it just breaks the skin before you core and stuff them.

Grapes 'n' Yogurt

Mix low-fat yogurt, a sprinkle of lemon juice and a dash of brown sugar. Stir in green or purple grapes. Chill and let flavours blend.

Hot Pear Delicacy

Sauté sliced, unpeeled pears in fruit juice. Add a pinch of cinnamon, nutmeg or ginger—your choice. Serve immediately with a scoop of fruit-flavoured sherbet.

Apricots on the BBQ

A terrific summer side dish. Just thread pitted fresh apricots on wooden skewers (which you've soaked for half an hour so they don't burn). Brush them lightly with a little melted brown sugar or honey and barbecue for about three minutes. Turn them over, baste them again and cook until soft.

Fruit-on-a-Stick

Made in seconds, this dessert is an easy way to encourage your family to eat more fruit. Simply skewer melon cubes and whole strawberries on a stick. Try bananas too, peach slices or halved plums. Whatever takes your fancy. Use low-fat vanilla yogurt as a dip.

Perfect Papaya Dressing

Easy enough to serve the family but fancy enough to wow your friends. Blend chunks of papaya and papaya seeds (yes, you can eat them) with the simple balsamic vinaigrette (see page 104). Toss it over a bowl of torn greens—the darker the better—and your salad is ready.

Frozen Bananas

My kids love these snack treats—and they're a great way to use your bananas if they've ripened before you're ready to eat them.

All you do is slice bananas into thick chunks, and freeze individually in plastic wrap. Eat frozen.

Moustache Drink

If mornings are crazy, drink breakfast! As delicious as a milkshake—but healthier.

Place a banana, half a cup of skim milk and a dash of vanilla in the blender. Add fresh or frozen fruit if you like. Buzz mixture for 30 seconds. Kids will love the moustache they get from drinking it.

TV Frozen Berries Treat

Picking ripe berries at a local farm is one of our favourite summer outings. We enjoy them right away, but we always freeze a bunch for winter nibbles. Just spread them on a cookie sheet in a single layer and leave in the freezer overnight. Then pop them in a plastic bag. They can last for months—although ours rarely do. Try them straight from the bag, or add them to the Moustache Drink. Too late to pick your own? You'll find summer's crop of raspberries, strawberries and blueberries in your supermarket freezer all year round.

Veggies and fruit at a glance

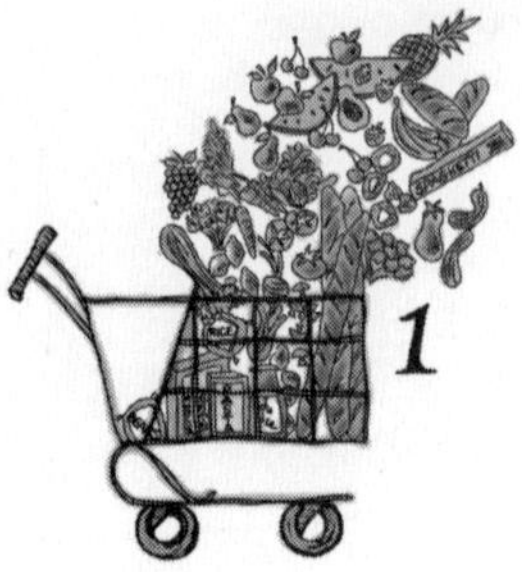

1

1. Fill your shopping cart with a variety of fruit and vegetables. They're rich in nutrients, a good source of fibre and most are low in fat.
2. Purchase locally grown fruit in season for peak freshness and best value.
3. Frozen fruit and vegetables are good choices when fresh produce is out of season.

Section 2 of your shopping cart

Milk Products

Meat and Alternatives

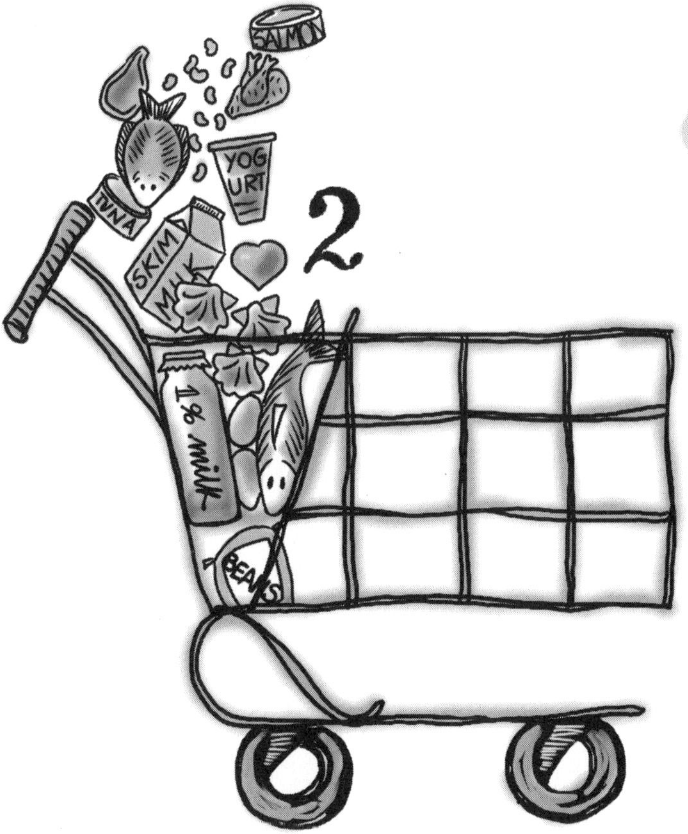

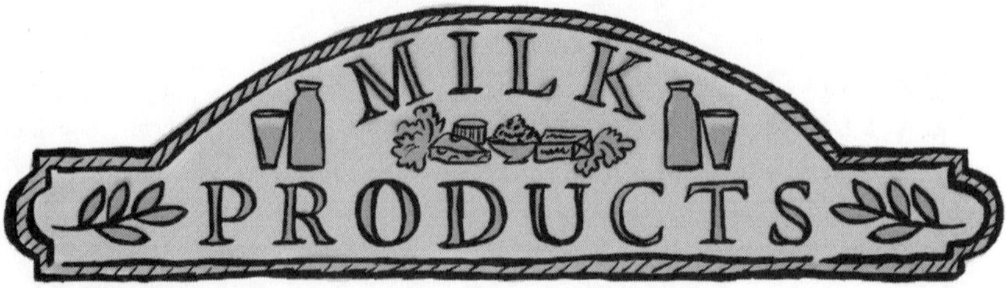

Be deliberate about how you fill the smaller #2 part of your cart, choosing lower-fat milk products.

Shopping cart shoppers, slow down. We're now in the #2 part of your cart, the milk products part, and here's where you have to think a little more carefully about what you choose. Milk is a highly nutritious food packed with vital nutrients essential for good health. Protein, carbohydrates, many vitamins and minerals, milk has a lot! Even when we get too grown-up for milk and cookies, it's still important that we get enough milk. But whole milk and products made from it also contain a lot of saturated fat and cholesterol. That's why they belong in the smaller #2 part of the HeartSmart shopping cart.

While it's fine to indulge in grains, vegetables and fruits to our heart's content, we need to take a slightly longer look at the milk products we pack in our cart. Fortunately, for the HeartSmart shopper, that's easy. Once the fat is skimmed, you have a HeartSmart choice. Take a good look through the dairy case and you'll find manufacturers have responded to our requests for lower-fat foods. These days, whole milk is far from being our only choice. Lower-fat varieties of milk, yogurt and cheese abound. By knowing some simple facts about milk products, we can make a dairy case for the best nutrition!

Milk: the big pitcher

Canada's Food Guide to Healthy Eating recommends at least 2 servings per day. But, depending on our age and stage in life, we may need more.

Children 4 - 9:	2-3 servings
Youth 10 - 16:	3-4 servings
Adults:	2-4 servings
Pregnant and breast-feeding women:	3-4 servings

One serving means:

- 1 cup (250 mL) milk
- 2 slices (50 g) processed cheese
- 1" x 1" x 3" (50 g) cheese
- 3/4 cup (175 mL) yogurt

Fat budgeting with milk products

Many milk products may be higher in fat, but lower-fat choices are widely available. That's why you need to think about fat budgeting before filling up the #2 part of your cart. Check the fat budget list and decide how you want to spend your fat budget.

fat Budget

Milk products:

0 tsp. fat	skim milk no-fat yogurt
1/2 tsp. fat	1 cup (250 mL) 1% milk 1 cup (250 mL) buttermilk
1 tsp. fat	2 tbsp (25 mL)parmesan cheese 1/4 cup (50 mL) low-fat ricotta 1 cup (250 mL) 2% milk 1 cup (250 mL) 2% cottage cheese
2 tsp. fat	1" x 1" x 3" (50 g) part-skim milk cheese 1/2 cup (125 mL) plain ice cream 1 cup (250 mL) whole milk 1 cup (250 mL) 4.5% cottage cheese
4 tsp. fat	1" x 1" x 3" (50 g) hard cheese

1 teaspoon fat = approximately 5 grams of fat.
These numbers are averages.

HeartSmart Tip

The fat in milk products is mostly saturated —a good reason to budget fat and choose the skimmed options.

fat Budget

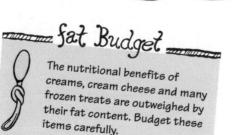

The nutritional benefits of creams, cream cheese and many frozen treats are outweighed by their fat content. Budget these items carefully.

To find out what nutrients milk products offer and where they fit in the total nutrition picture, see Appendix, page 124.

QA

What about milk and calcium?

Milk products are key sources of dietary calcium. We all need it, and women need it especially. Today one in four of us can expect to develop osteoporosis by the time we're 60. Consuming enough calcium helps build strong bones.

As well as calcium, milk contains vitamin D which helps calcium absorption. Milk also contains phosphorus which works with calcium to build bone.

ALL STAR TIP

Five steps to stave off osteoporosis

1. Consume enough calcium.
2. Do weight-bearing activities such as walking, hiking or dancing.
3. Get enough vitamin D.
4. Cut down on caffeine, salt and excessive protein.
5. Manage your weight—being underweight puts you at risk.

How much calcium is enough?

Adults need at least 1000 mg daily, and women need up to 1500 mg after menopause. If you are pregnant or nursing you should consume up to 1200 mg daily. Growing teens need a minimum 1200 mg.

Calcium? You've got it in the bag

Each of the following contains roughly 300 mg of calcium. Aim to have four servings daily—a total of 1200 mg.

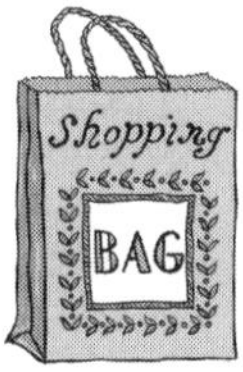

- 1 cup (250 mL) milk*
- 3/4 cup (175 mL) yogurt*
- 1 1/2 oz cheese (45 g)*
- 7 sardines with bones
- 1/2 - 3/4 can salmon with bones
- 1/2 cup (125 mL) almonds**
- 2 - 3 cups baked beans
- 1 1/2 cups (375 mL) sesame seeds**
- 3 cups (750 mL) broccoli
- 2 cups (500 mL) cottage cheese

*Choose skimmed versions whenever possible.
**While you can use almonds and sesame seeds to boost your calcium intake, they're too high in fat to be realistically considered as a source.

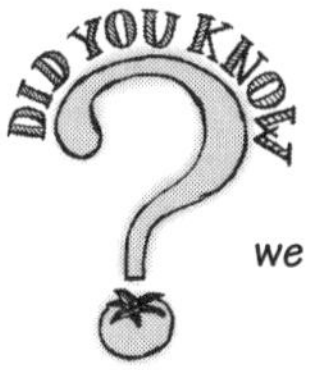

We drink half as much whole milk as we did 20 years ago.

Cutting fat without cutting milk

Thanks to the lower-fat milk products that abound, it's easy. Look for the % M.F. (milk fat) or % B.F. (butterfat) on the label and choose products with the lowest percentage of fat. Start by buying 2% instead of whole milk. Move down the fat scale to 1%. Try diluting 1% with skim for a week or two to gradually get yourself and your family used to skim milk.

Less fat doesn't mean less nutrition. You'll still be taking in all that valuable calcium. And by law milk must be fortified with fat-soluble vitamins A and D to replace any that are lost in the skimming process.

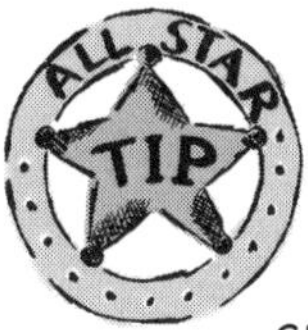

Don't leave milk products out of your diet because they're high in fat. Simply look for lower-fat options.

fat Budget

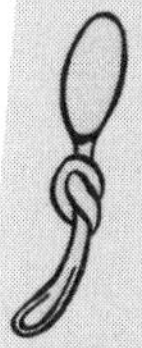

How much fat in a cup of milk?

0 tsp fat	skim milk
1/2 tsp fat	1%
1 tsp fat	2%
2 tsp fat	whole milk

Fat Budget

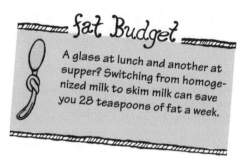

A glass at lunch and another at supper? Switching from homogenized milk to skim milk can save you 28 teaspoons of fat a week.

Did You Know

Milk math can be puzzling—2% milk actually contains 35% calories from fat. This is because the number refers to the percentage by weight, not calories, and much of the weight is water.

But don't be alarmed. While experts recommend a diet that derives no more than 30% calories from fat, this is a guide for your food intake over an entire day or even a week. It need not be applied to individual foods. Use percentages to compare products. When using milk, consider use. In tea or coffee, 2% milk is fine. You're only adding a spoonful or two. If you're pouring milk on your cereal or into a glass, 1% or skim milk are better choices.

All Star Tip

The percentage of fat that appears on a label usually refers to the percentage of fat by weight, not by calories. Use this percentage to compare products, not to judge the actual fat content.

Kidstuff

For the teen who *dislikes* milk

The problem is that your 15-year-old thinks milk is fattening. And, when you're growing up, you're often more concerned with how your body looks than what nutrients you're feeding it. Simply telling your son or daughter that milk is "good" for them probably won't work. Explaining the facts may.

Point out that they're making a great investment in their future health. Encourage them to consume skimmed dairy products which are low in fat and calories but loaded with nutrition. Mention that one glass of skimmed milk has only 80 calories—compared with the 140 calories in a bottle of pop.

Even if you're lactose-intolerant, there are still ways you can get the goodness of milk.

Add drops or tablets of lactase enzyme to your milk, or buy pretreated milk, or take pills containing the lactase enzyme.

Pick firm cheeses such as cheddar, edam and gouda which are virtually lactose free.

Choose yogurt or buttermilk, which contain live bacterial cultures that help you digest lactose more easily.

Try drinking milk "little and often" with meals throughout the day.

Tips to boost milk intake

- Add low-fat milk to soups instead of water.
- Make tasty drinks using low-fat milk as a base.
- Add powdered milk to soups and drinks.
- Make hot cereals with low-fat milk instead of water.

Which is better, bottles, cartons or pouches?

Nutritionally, there's no difference. Choose whichever you like.

Powdered, evaporated, sterilized, condensed...what's the difference?

Usually found in boxes near the flour and sugar in supermarkets, *skim milk powder* is a great low-fat choice. Keep some in your desk to add to your coffee if your office doesn't have a refrigerator. Add it to milkshakes, mashed potatoes, casseroles and cereals to bump up the nutrition. It has 70 mg of calcium per tablespoon and only 15 calories.

Available whole or skimmed, *canned evaporated milk* is handy to keep in your cupboard. It is found in the baking aisle as it's mostly used for baking. Evaporated milk is made by removing more than half the water in milk. It is fortified with vitamins A and D.

UHT milk is 2% milk treated at high temperatures. It can be stored at room temperature until opened and it still tastes like "real" milk.

Sweetened condensed milk at a whopping 1000 calories per cup breaks all the rules. As with evaporated milk, water is removed, but a large amount of sugar is added too.

A glass of milk will send you off to dreamland faster than counting sheep. It's not just an old wives' tale. Milk contains tryptophan, an amino acid that research has linked to helping us sleep. Try lower-fat milk with a teaspoon of honey and a dash of cinnamon.

What about goat's milk?

Tangy goat's milk contains most of the same nutrients as regular milk including lactose, but it is higher in fat, and you rarely find lower-fat versions. Some people think it is easier to digest than cow's milk, but there are no studies to prove this.

Do creams and non-dairy coffee lighteners belong in a HeartSmart cart?

Their fat content outweighs any nutritional benefits. Budget carefully.

KIDSTUFF

What about chocolate milk in the kids' lunchboxes?

Nutritionally, it's the same as ordinary milk. The milk is usually lower in fat — 2% or 1% milk fat (M.F.). But the chocolate syrup added, though low in fat, boosts the calories. You can make your own by adding chocolate milk mix or syrup to milk. If growing kids won't drink plain milk, give 'em chocolate milk.

Mystical magical yogurt

We've all heard the tales of Hunzas who live to be 120 years old and credit their age to a daily dose of yogurt. Cleopatra was said to have bathed in yogurt because it did wonderful things for her skin.

Promises, promises . . . Research shows that yogurt is useful in preventing and treating various intestinal problems such as diarrhea, but the nutritional truth is that yogurt is merely milk curdled by the addition of bacteria. It is certainly nutritious, but only as nutritious as its source, milk. It's an excellent source of calcium, protein and riboflavin but it may also hide fat and calories. Fortunately, your supermarket cooler is loaded with choices.

HeartSmart Tip

Check the fat. It's easy.

The yogurt container will tell you how much B.F. (butterfat) or M.F. (milk fat) it contains. The amount depends on which type of milk it is made from. It can range from a low 0.1 % (yogurt made from skim milk, 0 teaspoons fat) to as high as 10% (with added cream, 2 teaspoons fat). Select the lowest fat you can find, ideally 1% or less.

fat Budget

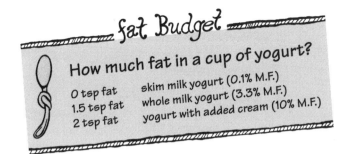

How much fat in a cup of yogurt?

0 tsp fat	skim milk yogurt (0.1% M.F.)
1.5 tsp fat	whole milk yogurt (3.3% M.F.)
2 tsp fat	yogurt with added cream (10% M.F.)

DID YOU KNOW

Sometimes the serving size described on a yogurt label is not consistent with the actual size of the container. Check the size if you're figuring out your fat intake.

KIDSTUFF

What about those drinkable yogurts that kids love?

A healthy choice for the lunchbox. Unfortunately, they can be pricey.

DID YOU KNOW

- Low-fat yogurt alert! It may not be as low in calories as you think. Adding fruit, fruit sauces or sundae ingredients adds calories. Read labels to compare products.
- Watch out for yogurt-covered nuts and raisins. Despite their name, these candies are not a good source of yogurt. The coating is merely a mixture of oil, sugar and yogurt powder.

ALL STAR TIP

Boost your yogurt intake

- Add yogurt to cold soup.
- Use yogurt as a base for veggie dips.
- Make yogurt salad dressings.

fun food...fast

Yummy yogurt ideas

Turn Yogurt into Cheese

Want the creaminess and richness of sour cream or cream cheese without the fat? Place low-fat yogurt in a cheesecloth-lined strainer over a bowl, or in a paper coffee filter in its holder. (Check that the yogurt doesn't contain gelatin or it won't strain.) Let it drain in the fridge to the consistency you want: a couple of hours for creamy, overnight for solid. Discard the whey that drips into the bowl. What remains is low-fat, versatile yogurt cheese, which can be used in so many ways.

Baked Potatoes

Top with yogurt cheese and chopped chives.

Vinaigrette

Substitute 2 parts yogurt cheese for 1 part oil.

Middle Eastern Bruschetta

Spread thin layer of yogurt cheese on toasted bread. Top with thinly sliced tomato, drizzle of olive oil and chopped mint.

Dessert

Sweeten yogurt or yogurt cheese with frozen fruit juice concentrates.

Fruit Dip

Mix 1 cup (250 mL) yogurt cheese with 1 tsp (5 mL) honey and a dash of cinnamon, grated nutmeg and grated orange rind.

Skinny Dipping with Yogurt

Low-fat yogurt or yogurt cheese makes a great dip. Simply use it in place of mayonnaise or sour cream in your favourite uncooked recipes. Low-fat yogurt plus:

- Mexican salsa
- Chopped fresh basil and onion
- Curry powder and chutney
- Honey mustard and dill (a pinch of sugar smooths out the flavour)

Surprise, it's buttermilk!

It sounds high in fat but it isn't. Buttermilk is usually made from lower-fat milk. Read the label.

fun food...fast

Buttermilk blasts

- Blend buttermilk with fresh fruit, sugar, vanilla and crushed ice for a delicious low-cal drink.
- Add tomato juice and a dash of cayenne or curry powder for a spicy drink.
- Drizzle over baked potatoes and top with fresh chives.
- Use as a base for cold summer soups.
- Swirl into hot soups at the last minute to enrich them.
- Use in sauces, salad dressing and mashed potatoes.

Be choosy with cheese

It takes 8 pounds of milk to make a pound of cheese. This super-concentrated food is a great source of calcium, but it's high in fat and calories too. A single ounce (30 grams) of hard cheese (the size of a domino) has about 300 mg calcium and 2 teaspoons fat.

fat Budget

How do you budget fat for cheese?

1 tsp fat	1 tbsp (15 mL) cream cheese
	2 tbsp (30 mL) parmesan
	1 oz (30 g) part-skim cheese (20% M.F. or less) (e.g., mozzarella)
	1/4 cup (50mL) lower-fat ricotta
	1 cup (250 mL) lower-fat cottage cheese (2%)
2 tsp fat	1 oz (30g) hard cheese (1" x 1" x 1/5") (e.g., American, cheddar, gouda, mozzarella, Swiss)
	1 cup (250 mL) creamed (4.5%) cottage cheese

ALL STAR TIP

You can lower the fat in your cheese choices by picking lower-fat cottage cheese or part-skim milk ricotta.

fat Budget

Choosing 1 ounce (30 g) part-skim mozzarella instead of 1 ounce cheddar cheese will save you 1 teaspoon of fat.

Q A

What about goat cheese?

Oops. While goat and sheep's milk cheeses are the rage with gourmets, they're not so popular with the HeartSmart crowd. The reason? High fat. Agreed, feta, Roquefort and chevre are delicious, but use them with caution. A better option? See if low-fat versions are available or use in small amounts.

DID YOU KNOW?

Vegetarians who substitute cheese for meat may be taking in more fat than they would like. Ounce for ounce, cheese has more calories, saturated fat, cholesterol and sodium than even the fattiest spareribs.

- LOW CHOLESTEROL or CHOLESTEROL-FREE cheese may not be low in fat. The butterfat may have been replaced by vegetable oil or the cheese may be a soy cheese. The amount of fat is the same but the type of fat is different.
- LOWER FAT may mean the cheese contains less fat than the original, but it still may not be low in fat.
- LOW CHOLESTEROL and LOW FAT cheeses are usually higher in sodium. Salt is added to compensate for the flavour that's lost when the fat is removed. Fat is essential to the taste and texture of cheese. Low-fat cheeses are less creamy and often less tangy.
- SOY CHEESE is still high in fat even though it has no cholesterol.

HeartSmart Tip

Use cheese as an extra for flavouring rather than eating chunks as a snack.

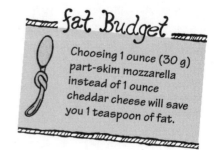

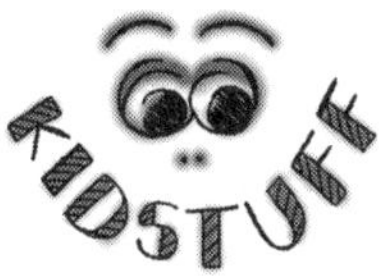

Kids love processed cheese

And it's so handy. Nutritionally, it is marginally lower in protein, vitamin A, calcium and iron, and higher in sodium.

Processed cheese is made by melting natural cheese with an emulsifier to form a smooth mass. Pasteurization helps these cheese foods keep longer. Check the label for added ingredients such as cream, and factor those into your buying decision.

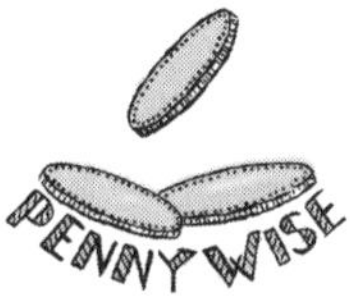

Always store cheese in foil. Plastic traps moisture which makes cheese mouldy. You can cut mould away from hard cheese but throw soft cheeses out. Mould may have penetrated deep beneath the surface.

We all scream for ice cream

Dutch chocolate, banana fudge, toffee maple . . . we all have our favourite frozen indulgence. And that's the best way to look at ice cream: as an occasional treat, not as part of your daily diet.

Real ice cream contains 10% milk by weight so ice cream is a good source of calcium with 100 – 150 mg per 1/2 cup (125 mL) serving. But usually it's high in saturated fat and calories too. If only it didn't taste so good . . .

The scoop on ice cream

Ice cream contains 1 to 2 teaspoons fat per 1/2 cup (125 mL). Gourmet ice creams may contain twice that amount!

Sherbet usually contains some dairy products as well as fruit.

Frozen dairy desserts such as ice milk are usually made with milk that is skimmed and are therefore lower in fat.

Frozen tofu desserts are dairy free, but they can be high in fat, even though the fat is mostly unsaturated.

Frozen yogurt is made like regular yogurt except that the culturing process is stopped before the characteristic tartness develops. Some varieties are low in fat, but others are made from cream or whole milk. Check the label.

Like it or not, broken cookies, sprinkles, nuts, chocolate chips and crumbled candy bars add extra fat, sugar and calories to your cone or sundae.

ALL STAR TIP

- Choose a frozen dessert containing less than 1 teaspoon of fat per ounce (5 g per 30 g). Regular ice cream has twice as much. Premium brands, even more. Keep serving size to 1/2 cup (125 mL) and enjoy it in balance.
- Fruit-based sorbets, fruit juice bars or fruit ices are an excellent choice. No fat. No cholesterol. Pick up a pack of moulds from the supermarket and make your own frozen treats for the family.

HeartSmart Tip Save almost 2 teaspoons of fat by choosing 1/2 cup sorbet (fruit ice) instead of 1/2 cup premium ice cream.

How much is enough?

When you're reading labels on frozen desserts, remember that a standard serving is 1/2 cup (125 mL)—which is probably less than you think. Measuring it out even once will give you a guideline to go by. Tricks to make it seem like more? Use smaller bowls or top each serving with fresh fruit.

Milk products at a glance

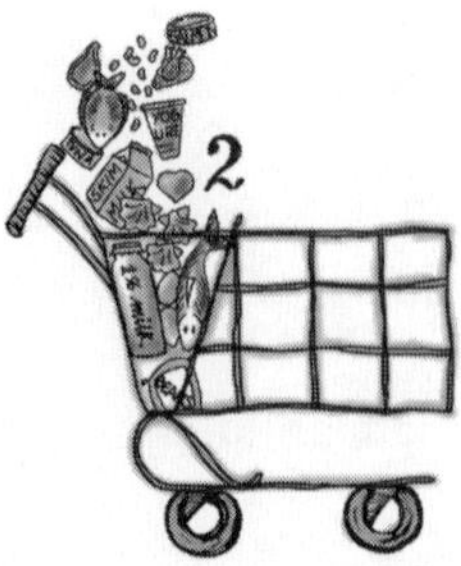

1. Look for milk products low in butterfat (B.F.) or milk fat (M.F.).
2. Choose milk, buttermilk, yogurt and cottage cheese with 2% or less B.F. or M.F.
3. Choose cheeses with 20% or less B.F. or M.F.

MEAT & ALTERNATIVES

Be deliberate about how you fill the #2 part of your cart, choosing lean meat, fish and legumes.

Time to slow down because here's where it gets a bit more complicated. Canada's Food Guide for Healthy Eating groups this eclectic range of foods together because they have one important nutrient in common: protein. But that's where the similarity ends.

Meat products—meat, poultry, fish, eggs—contain cholesterol but don't contain fibre. Plant products such as legumes and peanut butter have no cholesterol but do contain fibre. On top of that, each product has a different amount—and type—of fat. So how do you fill up this #2 part of your cart with nutrition smarts?

To cut the fat, especially the saturated fat, eat leaner meat in smaller portions. Make a little meat go a long way in stir-fries or pastas. Load up with deliciously versatile poultry, choosing white meat cuts with the skin removed. Go big on fish which is low in saturated fat and high in healthy omega-3s. Add lots of legumes—you won't be stuck for choice!

You may choose not to eat meat products at all for ethical, religious or environmental reasons. Your choice, but take time to ensure you get the balance you need of protein, iron, zinc and vitamin B12. Fill your cart with tasty meat alternatives such as beans, peas, lentils and tofu.

How much do we need?

Canada's Food Guide to Healthy Eating recommends two to three servings per day of meat, fish, eggs or alternatives.

One serving means:

1/3 cup (100 g) tofu	1/3–2/3 can (50g–100 g) canned fish
2 tbsp (30 mL) peanut butter	1/2–2/3 cup (125–150 mL) canned beans
50–100g meat, poultry or fish	1–2 eggs

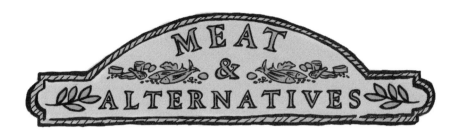

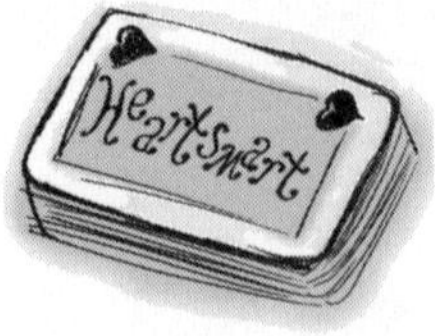

1 serving meat =
size of a deck of cards

Fat budgeting with meat and alternatives

Meat, fish, beans, eggs, nuts, seeds—so many options.

Check the fat budget lists below and decide how you want to spend your fat budget.

fat Budget

Meat and alternatives:

0 tsp. fat	dried beans (excluding soybeans), peas, lentils most white fish egg white
½ tsp. fat	90 g canned tuna in water 3 1/2 oz (100 g) skinless white chicken or turkey
1 tsp. fat	1 tbsp (15 mL) nuts or seeds 1 medium egg 1 slice (25 g) salami 1 small sausage 3 1/2 oz (100 g) tofu (amount of fat differs, depending on firmness; check label) 3 1/2 oz (100 g) skinless dark chicken or turkey 3 1/2 oz (100 g) lean beef, pork, lamb 1 cup (250 mL) chickpeas 1 cup (250 mL) soy drink
2 tsp. fat	1 small wiener 3 1/2 oz (100 g) canned salmon 3 1/2 oz (100 g) white chicken or turkey with skin 3 1/2 oz (100 g) beef, pork, lamb 3 1/2 oz (100 g) extra lean ground beef

3 tsp. fat

2 tbsp peanut butter
3 1/2 oz (100 g) dark chicken or turkey with skin
3 1/2 oz (100 g) lean ground beef
1 cup (250 mL) cooked soybeans

4 tsp. fat

3 1/2 oz (100 g) salami
3 1/2 oz (100 g) regular ground beef
3 1/2 oz (100 g) ribs

1 teaspoon fat = approximately 5 grams of fat.
These numbers are averages.

HeartSmart Tip Choose beans and fish more often because they're lower in saturated fat.

To find out what nutrients are in meat and alternatives and where they fit in the total nutrition picture, see Appendix, page 124.

Meat: cut it down—no need to cut it out

It's not meat itself that's the problem, it's eating fatty cuts and eating too much of them. It's all about balance.

The concern about meat is the total fat and saturated fat, which are linked to an increased risk of heart disease.

No question, the trend today is to eat less meat. How times have changed. It used to be that a meal wasn't a meal unless it was meat and potatoes—a big hunk of meat was regarded as a status symbol. In fact, North Americans have always tended to eat more meat than other nations. In countries where meat is expensive, it's regarded more as a condiment and the bulk of the plate is filled with vegetables and grains.

The trend towards eating less red meat is based nutritionally on a sound concern about fat, especially saturated fat. But while we don't need nearly as much meat—or protein—as we've grown used to eating, make no mistake—meat does supply important nutrients.

ALL STAR TIP

- Eating foods high in dietary cholesterol will not necessarily raise your blood cholesterol, but if your blood cholesterol is high, cut down on your intake of dietary cholesterol (see Appendix).
- Treat meat as a side dish that complements a meal of veggies, grains or legumes.
- Avoid eating organ meats (e.g., liver and kidney) where cholesterol and contaminants may be concentrated.

DID YOU KNOW

We are eating less red meat than ever. Consumption of meat has dropped almost 30% since the mid-seventies—and almost one in seven of us has cut out meat completely.

Large amounts of meat don't make you stronger. You can only achieve that by exercising your muscles against resistance. Lift weights, not steaks.

Lean meat shortcuts

The fat content in meat isn't labelled. These few simple tips will help you make lower-fat choices in the meat department.

Use your eyes

Look for the leanest meat you can. Cut off all visible fat. The fat you can see marbling some meat cuts—those white streaks—is impossible to remove. Choose those cuts rarely.

Check its speedometer

I'm serious. If an animal can move faster than you, it's lean. Buffalo (bison), deer (venison), rabbit, partridge, pheasant and quail—choose any one of these and you'll win out nutritionally. A lower percentage of fat. Lower in cholesterol. Plus more intense flavour so you'll be satisfied with less. Talk about a win-win situation.

Test your meat cut IQ

Meat from close to the ribs has the most fat. It's logical. The animal needs a fatty layer to protect its vital organs from injury. Cuts to limit are short-ribs, whole ribs and blade roast. Cuts of meat close to the hip usually have the least fat. These areas are on the move. They can take care of themselves. Good choices are cuts such as sirloin tip roast and steaks, eye of the round and tenderloin.

Deal yourself a HeartSmart serving
The size of a deck of cards is about right.

HeartSmart Tip Meat cuts with the words "round" or "loin" on the label are lean. Good choices.

DID YOU KNOW Lean ground beef is not necessarily as low in fat as lean cuts of meat.

ALL STAR TIP Decrease the fat content of ground beef before adding it to chili or spaghetti by browning in a nonstick pan and draining the fat.

fat Budget

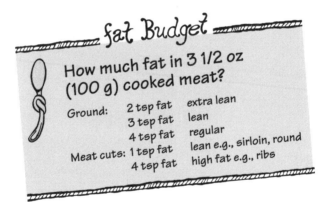

How much fat in 3 1/2 oz (100 g) cooked meat?

Ground:	2 tsp fat	extra lean
	3 tsp fat	lean
	4 tsp fat	regular
Meat cuts:	1 tsp fat	lean e.g., sirloin, round
	4 tsp fat	high fat e.g., ribs

QA *What if the meat looks purple?*
Meat is red from the myoglobin it contains (an oxygen-storing muscle pigment) not from blood, most of which is removed when the animal is slaughtered. The harder the muscle has worked, the darker the meat colour. That's why chicken and turkey legs are dark while wings and breasts are white.

Meat that is not exposed to oxygen (such as the inside of a roast, or vacuum-packed meat) is dark purple. It needn't affect your choice.

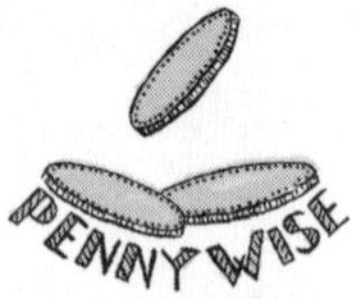

Best meat for your money

- Check the "best before" date on the label. Often meat close to that date is reduced in price. Use the same day.
- Look for cream-coloured fat that springs when you touch it. Avoid, hard yellow fat. Remove all fat once you get it home.
- Exposure to oxygen turns meat brown. It's still edible but you should use it immediately.

In general, today's meat is leaner. Ranchers are crossbreeding lean with traditional breeds and sending cattle to market younger—and leaner.

More fat is trimmed away at the packing stage before the meat reaches the market.

Pork picks

Pork is leaner than it used to be, and low-fat cuts can be compared to the leanest cuts of beef. Pork fat is lower in saturated fat than beef fat—but it's still not as lean as skinless turkey or chicken breast.

Choose lean cuts with the word "loin" such as tenderloin, center loin, top loin, lean ham or fresh pork leg.

Limit fattier cuts like spareribs, bacon, ground pork or shoulder roast.

Keep portions to the size of a deck of cards.

If you are watching your salt intake, limit bacon, ham and cold cuts.

Choosing lamb?

Lean cuts are more tender than similar cuts of beef. Leanest cut? Leg of lamb.

HeartSmart Tip

Home Test

Not sure how much saturated fat a meat contains? Here's an easy way to find out.

Next time you cook red meat, refrigerate leftovers overnight. The following morning look at the fat on top. It's white, hard, and you can crack it with a knife. This is saturated fat, the kind that encourages arteries to clog up with plaque and slows down blood flow.

Try the same test with cooked chicken. You'll see that the fat is softer in texture since it has less saturated fat. The fat found in fish is oily, since it is a polyunsaturated fat.

A reminder: if chilled fat looks as though it could block up your sink, it might block up your arteries too.

Meat is made of iron

Meat is full of iron—the kind that is more readily absorbed by the body than that found in legumes. Women especially need to be on the watch for iron deficiency. We need to make special efforts to obtain enough iron from our diet. Meat is also a good source of zinc and vitamin B12. If you cut out animal foods, eat lots of legumes, whole grains leavened with yeast, and processed soy products to supply zinc—and take a vitamin B12 supplement.

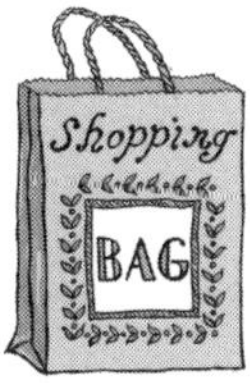

Plants armed with iron

- LEGUMES: *dried peas, bean curd (tofu), kidney beans, lima beans*
- GRAINS AND CEREAL: *enriched or fortified products eg. breakfast cereal (cream of wheat, oatmeal), breads, spaghetti*
- FRUITS: *dried apricots, raisins, prunes*
- VEGETABLES: *broccoli, bok choy, beet greens*
- OTHERS: *almonds, sesame seeds, blackstrap molasses*

Ironclad tips on plant sources

Iron is better absorbed from animal than vegetable sources, and some vegetables contain substances that hinder absorption. Tables listing the iron content of plant foods only tell half the story.

To increase absorption:

- Consume a vitamin C-containing food (such as a glass of orange juice) with your iron source.
- Eat a small amount of meat or fish at the same time.
- Avoid drinking black or green tea with iron-containing plant sources.
- Cook in cast iron pots.

Cluck-cluck!

Poultry used to be a special Sunday dinner treat. Not any more. Changes in breeding and marketing techniques mean that it's more abundant and affordable than ever. In fact, Canada produces more chicken in 24 hours than was produced in the whole of one year in the 1930s.

Add it to your HeartSmart shopping cart and enjoy its versatility—who ever gets tired of eating chicken? Choose turkey too, which is even lower in fat. Not all parts of chicken are low in total fat. Eating the skin more than doubles the amount of fat and saturated fat.

HeartSmart Tip Chicken has roughly the same amount of cholesterol as red meat but is lower in fat, and the fat is less saturated.

Guide to buying poultry

ALL STAR TIP

- Choose white rather than dark meat to get less fat and a little less cholesterol.
- Look for moist, plump poultry—that means it's fresh—and give it a sniff. It should smell clean.
- Frozen poultry should be rock hard. Ice crystals or frozen liquid mean that it has been defrosted and then re-frozen. The result? Loss of flavour.
- Buy ground poultry from a reputable butcher. Sometimes skin is mixed in which makes it higher in fat than ground beef.

fat Budget

How much fat in half a breast or a whole leg of chicken (3 1/2 oz or 100 g)?

1/2 tsp fat	light meat, no skin
2 tsp fat	with skin
1 tsp fat	dark meat, no skin
3 tsp fat	with skin

* Measurements are approximate. Turkey has slightly less fat than chicken.

Turning to turkey

Lower in fat than chicken, turkey is an excellent HeartSmart choice. Almost all turkey fat is found in the skin. Just cut it away.

Substitute ground turkey in your favourite ground beef recipes such as burgers or meatballs. Just add bread crumbs, egg white, Worcestershire sauce and mustard.

HeartSmart Tip

Choose 3 1/2 ounces (100 g) light meat without any skin instead of 3 1/2 ounces dark meat with skin and you'll save 2 1/2 teaspoons of fat.

Chicken wings are mostly skin (and a chicken's fat is under its skin). Limit how many you eat.

DID YOU KNOW

How to size up a chicken

You can tell the approximate age of a chicken by pressing against the breast-bone. If it's pliable, it's young and tender.

Most chickens sold in the supermarket are broilers (sometimes called fryers). Weighing between 2.5 and 5 pounds (1.2-2.2 kg), they can be roasted, grilled, steamed, sautéed, poached, broiled or fried.

Roasting chickens are big guys, older and larger chickens that weigh up to 6 pounds (2.7 kg). Perfect for a family-sized roast chicken dinner.

PENNY WISE

Boneless chicken breast is no more expensive, ounce for ounce than bone-in. But if you're handy with a knife, buy bone-in and use the bones for stock.

Think twice at the deli counter

Fast for sandwiches, quick in salads, deli meats are the ultimate in convenience. But they're not perfect. In fact they may pack a double whammy of substances that you might not want to feed your family: fat and sodium.

fat Budget

Hard facts on cold cuts

Cut down on high-fat cold cuts such as bologna, salami, side bacon, sausages, wieners, liverwurst and pâté. Choose turkey breast, pastrami and low-fat ham with less than 1 gram of fat—only a fraction of a teaspoon—per ounce.

Many popular cold cuts now come in a turkey version—but they're not as lean as turkey breast. Dark meat is often used and some cuts contain turkey hearts and gizzards which are high in cholesterol and fat. Turkey roll, bologna and salami may be as high in fat as versions made from beef.

HeartSmart Tip Limit favourite deli accompaniments such as pickles, olives and sauerkraut. They're high in salt.

The sizzle on sausages

Most sausages are pork based, but they can be made from any kind of chopped ground meat. It's the seasoning that gives Italian sausage or Mexican chorizo its distinctive flavour. Most sausages are high in fat and sodium. They may contain 2 to 3 teaspoons of fat depending on size. But you may find lower-fat sausages occasionally. Read the labels and watch that fat budget.

The hot news on hot dogs

Beef, pork, chicken, turkey or tofu—whichever kind you pick, do your homework first. Read the label to check the fat content and keep the following info in mind:

Chicken or turkey dogs may not necessarily be low in fat. If they're made from dark meat and skin, their fat content will be high.

Tofu hot dogs may be leaner and they do offer a nutritional advantage—the fat they contain is unsaturated and they have no cholesterol.

Beware of claims that hot dogs are 90% fat free. This is a measure of fat by weight, not by calories. Check the label to find out the fat content.

fat Budget

Hot diggity dog! Lower-fat hot dogs contain less than 1 teaspoon fat. Regular dogs have two or three times as much.

Reel in some fish

Seafood is good for you. All kinds. Both fish and shellfish are low in fat and saturated fat. Any fats contained in fish are the healthy omega-3 fatty acids (see Appendix, page 126) which may protect you against heart disease. Most varieties (except for shrimp, squid and caviar) are low in cholesterol too. Load up the #2 part of your shopping cart.

Hook the best

Check packaging for the "best before" date.

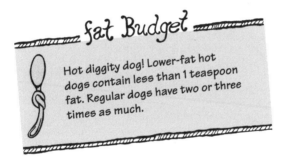

Buy fish last on your trip and store it in its original wrapper in the coldest part of your refrigerator (under the freezer or in the meat container).

Choose steaks and fillets that are moist. Whole fish should have red or bright pink gills and shiny, tightly clinging scales.

Throw fish back if...

- it smells fishy
- it's brown or dry around the edges
- it's covered with ice crystals or has freezer burn

ALL STAR TIP

- Eat fish at least two to three times a week.
- Avoid eating skin, which is where fat and contaminants may be concentrated.

fun food...fast

Fish made fabulous

Plain, simple fish is the perfect low-fat choice for a healthy meal. Bake, broil or grill, adding flavour with herbs and lemon or orange juice. Spicy salsas add zest.

To cook whole fish, measure at its thickest part and cook for 10 minutes for every inch. Fish is cooked when it's opaque. Salmon, which is higher in fat than other fish, can be cooked longer without drying out.

To microwave, place fish in microwaveable dish. Season with pepper, lemon juice or herbs (do not add salt until after cooking). Cover with plastic wrap, leaving one corner open to get rid of steam. Cook until fish flakes when tested with a fork.

fat Budget

Fatty fish, lean fish, they're all HeartSmart. How much fat in 3 1/2 oz (100 g) fresh fish?

0 tsp fat	cod, flounder, haddock, monkfish, pike, pollock, perch, whiting, red snapper, halibut, sole
1 tsp fat	swordfish, fresh bluefin tuna, trout
2 tsp fat	salmon, albacore, mackerel, herring, bluefish, sardines

DID YOU KNOW

- The fat in fatty fish is largely unsaturated. It's high in omega-3 fatty acids and it's thought that this fat may help protect our hearts and blood flow. Feel free to feast on high-fat fish, but check your fat budget.
- The rumours are false! With the exception of shrimp, shellfish are *not* significantly high in cholesterol. While they do contain some, the amount is often no higher than chicken or beef (see Appendix, page 127). They are low in fat and a good option—provided you don't serve melted butter on the side.

HeartSmart Tip Canned fish provides the same health benefits as fresh fish. Choose water- or broth-packed fish or drain the oil from oil-packed fish.

fat Budget

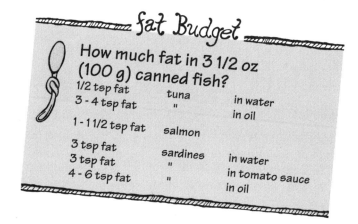

How much fat in 3 1/2 oz (100 g) canned fish?

1/2 tsp fat	tuna	in water
3 - 4 tsp fat	"	in oil
1 - 1 1/2 tsp fat	salmon	
3 tsp fat	sardines	in water
3 tsp fat	"	in tomato sauce
4 - 6 tsp fat	"	in oil

HeartSmart Tip A 3 1/2 oz can of oil-packed tuna contains 3 to 4 teaspoons of fat before you drain it. Why not choose water-packed tuna instead?

ALL STAR TIP

Boost your calcium intake by eating the bones of canned sardines and salmon.

What about imitation shellfish?

They look like their wealthier crab and lobster cousins but how do these look-alikes cut it nutritionally? The answer is, very well. They're a tasty addition to salads and sandwiches and, at only 100 calories for 3 1/2 ounces (100 g), a wise choice if you're watching your weight.

These pretenders are made mainly from pollock, a deep-sea whitefish which is low in fat and rich in high-quality protein. The filleted fish is ground, then refined to remove its natural color, flavour and odour. New colour and flavour are added. The results are crab legs, shrimp, scallops and lobster tails that resemble the real thing.

The differences? Imitation shellfish has more sodium and less omega-3 fatty acid. Processing destroys some of the vitamins and minerals.

Where do fish sticks fit?

Be wary. With their batter coating they contain more fat and salt than fresh fish. If you serve them with ketchup and cocktail sauce you also raise your sodium intake. Tartar sauce adds extra fat too. See page 120.

Cracking the case for eggs

Egg consumption dropped by over 20% between 1980 and 1990 as North Americans became cholesterol-conscious. Turns out you may not need to cut down on the eggs you eat.

Eggs are a powerhouse of nutrition, and rich in protein, B vitamins, vitamin A and iron. They're economical too, and you can't beat them for versatility.

People are often concerned that eggs are a major source of cholesterol. It's true. A single egg contains about 210 mg dietary cholesterol as well as 1 teaspoon of fat. But remember, it's not so much the cholesterol as the saturated fat in your diet that affects your blood cholesterol. An egg contains less than half a teaspoon of saturated fat (compared with 1 teaspoon in a 3 1/2 ounce [100 g] hamburger patty).

ALL STAR TIP

Egg whites don't contain fat or cholesterol. Eat as much as you like. You can successfully switch two egg whites for one whole egg in most recipes—or substitute one whole egg and two egg whites for two whole eggs.

PENNYWISE

Buying and storing eggs safely

Never purchase eggs that have been sitting at room temperature. Always buy refrigerated eggs, and pop them in the fridge when you get home—not in the egg rack where they are exposed to warm air each time you open the fridge, but on the shelf in their original carton.

Avoid eggs with visible cracks. Before you lift a carton into your cart, jiggle each egg to make sure that it's not stuck to the bottom. It takes time but it's worth it.

QA

Should I limit the eggs I eat?

Maybe. Maybe not.

Most people can eat eggs in moderation without any harmful effects on their blood cholesterol. But limit your intake to two eggs a week if you or your family have high blood cholesterol. You don't have to limit the number of egg whites you use.

Brown eggs or white eggs?

Yolk and shell colour have no bearing on an egg's nutritional quality.

What about egg substitutes?

Made from egg whites, with vegetable oil, flavour and coloring added, these are not necessarily low in fat. The equivalent of one egg may contain as much as 4 grams, almost 1 teaspoon. But the fat is unsaturated and they are cholesterol free.

How can I avoid leftover egg yolks?

Check your supermarket cooler for egg whites available in liquid form. These make a good substitute for fresh eggs and save you the task of separating the yolk from the white—and they spare you the problem of what to do with all those yolks.

Meet the legendary legume family

As we continue to fill the #2 part of our shopping cart, it's time to look at legumes (dried beans, peas and lentils). While they fit happily within the meat group because they are high in protein, their family background is vegetarian.

Legumes are simply the seeds that grow inside the pods of leguminous plants. We know them mostly as dried beans, peas and lentils. A poor man's meat? No way! Inexpensive, yes, but legumes are crammed with nutrition. Consider what they offer. Soluble fibre for starters—the kind that may reduce blood cholesterol. Loads of B vitamins, lots of protein and little fat. To cap it off, they're also a source of calcium, iron and potassium.

They're also versatile and very, very cheap. In truth, they would fit well in the #1 part of your shopping cart.

One cup (250 mL) of most legumes = 200 to 300 calories and 6 to 12 grams fibre.

Are legumes a good source of protein?

Legumes are almost perfect—but not quite. They lack one or more amino acids (protein building blocks). All you do is add the missing amino acid, which you'll find in other grains, nuts, seeds or in small amounts of animal foods. Don't even worry about having to eat both at the same meal. As long as they are eaten over the course of the day you'll be doing fine nutritionally.

Buying and cooking peas, beans and lentils

Supermarkets carry a growing range of legumes. You'll find them available dried or canned. With both kinds on hand, you're equipped to make dozens of flavourful dishes. Cook up a big batch of beans at a time and freeze them for future use. Caution: canned beans can have added salt. You may want to rinse them under cold running water.

There are three ways to prepare dried legumes for cooking. Always start by rinsing them well:

- Soak them overnight, adding 3 parts of water for 1 part beans. Discard soaking water before cooking.
- Add beans to water and bring to a boil. Let boil for 2 minutes, remove from heat and let stand for an hour. Discard soaking water before cooking.
- Combine beans and water in a microwaveable dish. Cover and microwave at full power for 15 minutes or until boiling. Let stand one hour. Drain.

Beans, beans, the musical fruit...

We all know about those unfortunate side effects. Soaking beans well and cooking them in fresh water will help to get rid of some of the sugars that produce gas.

Bean around the world?

Maybe the budget won't stretch to a trip to Europe or Mexico, but beans can take your tastebuds there. Legumes have been a part of diets world-wide for thousands of years. Even today, they are a dietary staple of billions. Think of Mexican tamales and bean burritos, Indian dahl, Middle Eastern hummus and falafel, Cuban black beans and rice, Italian minestrone soup, Chinese bean curds and bean sprouts—all dishes guaranteed to brighten up your dinner plate.

Compared with fresh beans or peas, dried varieties have more concentrated protein and other nutrients—enough in fact to grow a whole new plant.

The no-cook good news

You don't have to start from scratch. Good news if you're off to the store and supper has to be on the table in an hour. Use canned legumes instead. Black beans, white beans, red beans, lentils—you'll find them all on the shelf waiting to be packed in your cart and turned into something wonderful for supper. Just drain and rinse (to reduce any excess salt) and add to your favourite recipe.

Green, red, yellow or brown, lentils need no soaking. They take just 10 to 30 minutes to cook. Think of them as the express-lane legume.

fun food...fast

Bean salad

3 cups (750 mL) canned (or cooked) beans
1/2 cup each (125 mL) chopped green and red peppers and onion
1/4 cup (50 mL) low-calorie salad dressing

Toss together and enjoy.

What about soybeans?

Evidence is emerging that soybeans, a member of the legume family, and some soy products might help prevent—and even fight—cancer because of the phytochemicals they contain (see page 46 for more on phytochemicals).

They have been a staple and an important source of protein in Asia for over five thousand years. Buy them prebagged or in bulk and store in an air-tight container.

DID YOU KNOW

Soybeans are different from other beans

- The only vegetable food that contains a complete protein
- Both soluble and insoluble fibre
- The only bean that contains fat. Soybean "fat" is mostly unsaturated and might help lower blood cholesterol levels.

A soybean feast

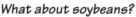

Soy doesn't just mean beans. It's the starting point for miso, soynuts, soy sauce, tempeh, tofu and TVP. Not sure which is which? Here's the scoop on soy products.

Miso	The term for a number of rich, salty condiments, indispensable to Japanese cooking. Store miso in the refrigerator and use sparingly because of salt content.
Soynuts	Roasted whole soybeans. Look for the dry-roasted variety. These crunchy high-protein snacks are higher in fat if they have been oil-roasted.
Soy sauce	A mixture of soybeans, wheat flour and yeast which has been

fermented for about 18 months. The liquid is extracted and then processed. Use sparingly because of salt content.

Tempeh Fermented soybeans make this traditional Indonesian food, which has a stronger flavour than tofu. You'll generally find it in the frozen foods case.

Tofu A bland, soft, cheeselike food, tofu is made by curdling fresh hot soy milk with either nigari—a compound found in ocean water—or the compound calcium sulfate. The curds are then shaped and pressed into blocks. Because it's rich in protein and iron, the Chinese call it "meat without bones" and use it extensively in their cooking. Check the label. If the calcium salt has been used to curdle it, it's rich in calcium too.

Tofu soaks up flavours like a sponge. It's easy and fast to prepare and easy to digest—and it doesn't cause gas! Firm tofu can replace meat in stir-fry dishes, soups or on the grill. It has more protein, calcium and fat than other forms of tofu. Try soft tofu in Asian soups.

You'll find fresh tofu in the produce, dairy or deli sections. It's also sold in deep-fried strips and pouches. You can buy fresh tofu in vacuum packs, in water-filled tubs or in aseptic brick packages. The packaged kind have a "best before" date. You can store the tofu varieties sealed in liquid. Once they are opened, drain off the water and replace water daily. Use within a week.

TVP (Textured Soy Protein) When soy flour is compressed, its protein fibres change in structure and its texture becomes similar to ground beef. TVP is often used to extend products such as meats. It has a long shelf life because it is low in moisture.

Nuts and seeds

A wonderful snack, in moderation. Nuts and seeds balance the protein in other vegetable foods and can be a nourishing snack on hiking or camping trips. Just remember, eat them one by one, not by the handful.

fat Budget

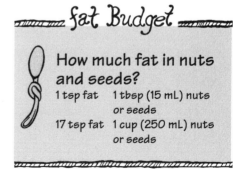

How much fat in nuts and seeds?

1 tsp fat	1 tbsp (15 mL) nuts or seeds
17 tsp fat	1 cup (250 mL) nuts or seeds

DID YOU KNOW?

Dry-roasted peanuts contain all the fat of the original nut. Enjoy as an occasional treat. Roasted peanuts are fried in oil.

Shell out for peanut butter

One, it's a good protein substitute. Two, it's a bargain. Peanut butter is simply peanuts ground into a paste. A staple in many homes, it's high in protein and that's why it's in the #2 part of your cart. It is rich in minerals and vitamin B but watch the fat content.

fat Budget

2 tbsp (25 mL) peanut butter = 3 tsp fat.

ALL STAR TIP

- Making peanut butter sandwiches? You don't need to add butter or margarine.
- Shop wisely. Choose peanut butter that isn't laced with sugar, salt and hydrogenated vegetable oil.
- To prevent non-hydrogenated peanut butter from separating, heat in microwave for a couple of minutes and stir .
- Once opened, store peanut butter in the fridge, especially unhomogenized types made from 100% ground peanuts. Throw out a jar that has gone mouldy.

Meat and alternatives at a glance

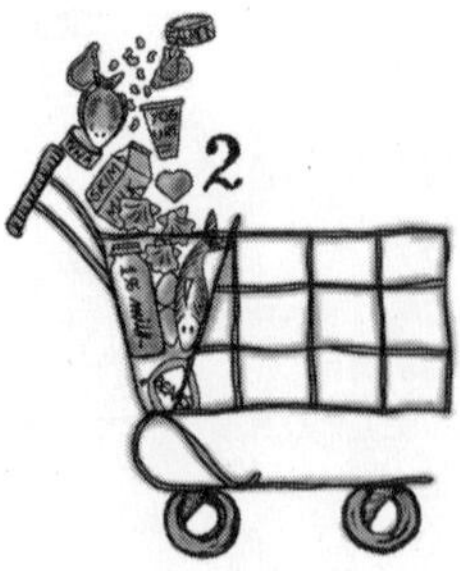

1. Choose lean cuts, trim visible fat and remove skin from poultry.
2. Choose fish more often.
3. Load up on beans, peas and lentils.

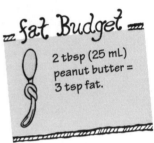

Section 3 of your shopping cart

Fats, Oils and Others

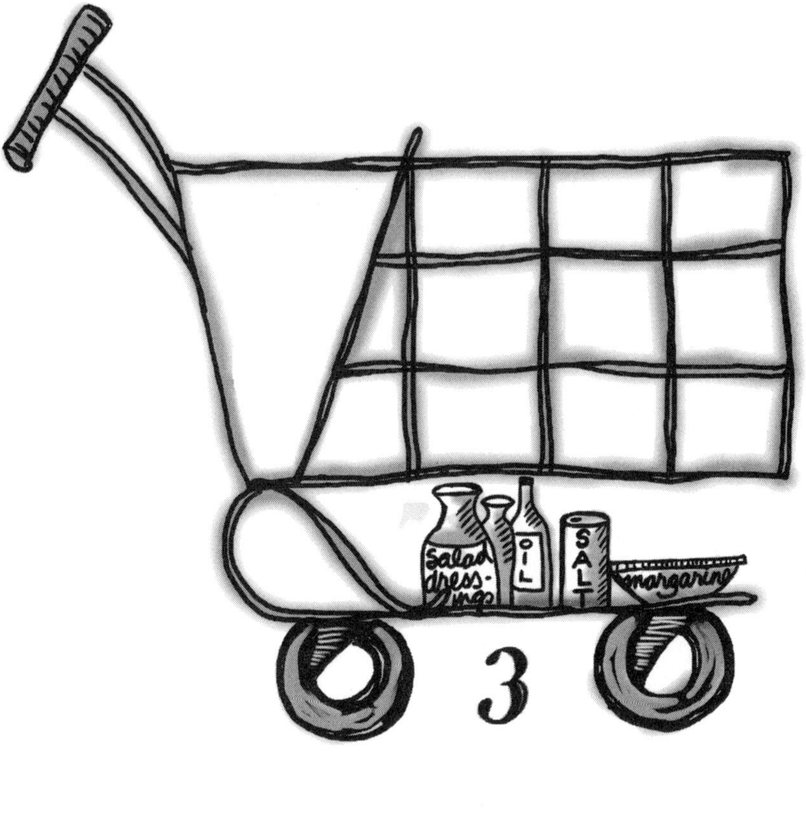

FATS, OILS & OTHERS

Think carefully about what you add to the #3 lower part of your cart. The less fat the better.

Now we get to the #3 part of your shopping cart—the other side of the nutrition rainbow. Be frugal here . . . seriously. You won't see these foods on the rainbow even though they're in Canada's Food Guide to Healthy Eating, because many of them offer too much fat relative to their nutritional value.

We're on the right track. Most of us make a real effort to cut back on animal fats, but that's only part of the story. As we're reducing our fat consumption by choosing lower-fat meat and milk products, we've increased our intake of vegetable oils, some of which are saturated or hydrogenated. Today, on average, we eat 50% of fat in the form of cooking oils, margarine, salad dressings, baked goods and fried foods. Too much! That's why this part of your shopping cart calls for a very careful look. Fats, oils and others do fit—but choose wisely. Think lower. Think frugal.

Fat budgeting with fats, oils and others

Look for lower-fat and no-fat versions of these foods. New ones are appearing every day. Check the fat-budget list and decide how you want to spend your fat budget.

fat Budget

Fats, oils and others:

0 tsp. fat	fat-free salad dressing fat-free mayonnaise

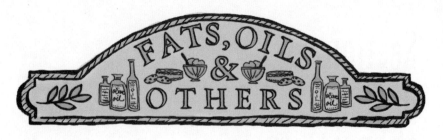

1 tsp. fat

1 tsp (5 mL) oil, cooking or salad
1 tsp (5 mL) butter
1 tsp (5 mL) margarine
2 tsp (5 mL) low-fat margarine
1 tbsp (15 mL) low-fat mayonnaise
1 tbsp (15 mL) cream cheese
1 tbsp (15 mL) cheese spread
2 tbsp (30 mL) sour cream
2 tbsp (30 mL) half-and-half
2 tbsp (30 mL) whipping cream
2 tbsp (30 mL) shredded coconut

2 tsp. fat

1 tbsp (15 mL) salad dressing
1 tbsp (15 mL) mayonnaise
15 chips — potato, corn, nacho

3 tsp. fat

1 small 50g chocolate bar, plain

1 teaspoon fat = approximately 5 grams of fat.
These numbers are averages.

HeartSmart Tip

Many products found in this section have labels stating the grams of fat they contain. Just remember that 5 g fat = approximately 1 tsp fat.

ALL STAR TIP

- Try nut butters or non-hydrogenated margarine instead of butter or hydrogenated margarine.
- Read labels and choose processed products in which the unsaturated fat is NOT hydrogenated.

We need to eat some fat

Fat plays an important role in overall nutrition.

- It carries the fat-soluble vitamins, A, D, E and K.
- It's a concentrated source of energy.

- It gives a glow to our skin and a shine to our hair.
- It helps us feel full by keeping food in the stomach longer.
- It provides the essential fatty acids which our bodies can't make and which we must get from foods.

Keeping your eye on visible fat

Some fats you can see, some you can't. Visible fat is the fat you can see, or the fat you buy to add to your food. Oils, margarines, butter, salad dressings, nuts, seeds, cream and coffee whiteners all come under this category.

Oils

All oils are 100% fat and the same number of calories as solid fats. The difference is the type of fat. You may find you're confused by what's on the label. A couple of explanations:

No cholesterol doesn't mean that the oil is special. All oils are vegetable products, so they don't contain cholesterol anyway. Manufacturers could just as well put "no diamond dust" on the label. If you want to reduce your blood cholesterol you need to reduce your total fat intake. All oils are 100% fat.

Light doesn't mean that the oil is light in fat or calories. "Light" usually refers to lightness of texture, flavour or colour.

DID YOU KNOW

Oils sold in supermarkets are high in unsaturated fat. The tropical oils—palm, palm kernel and coconut oil—which are high in saturated fat, are not sold commercially but are used in many processed products.

HeartSmart Tip

While all oils sold in supermarkets are high in unsaturated fat, none of them are 100% unsaturated. The solution? Try to use as little as possible.

fat Budget

All oils are 100% fat.

How to add less oil to your food

ALL STAR TIP

- When you're cooking with oil, try to use nonstick pans and heat the oil before you add the food. That way, the food sits in the oil for a shorter time and absorbs less.
- Using mellow balsamic or fruit vinegars in salad dressings lets you use less oil. Mustard, herbs and garlic will also boost the flavour.
- Spray your baking pans with a cooking spray that contains vegetable oil (such as corn or soy) plus lecithin which helps oil and water solutions stick together. These sprays prevent sticking by forming a thin film between the food and the baking tray. Shake the can well before using and use only on cold surfaces.

QA

Are olive oils and canola oil HeartSmart choices?

Yes, because they're high in monounsaturates. This does not mean that more is better. All oil is still 100% fat. Remember your fat budget!

DID YOU KNOW?

Olive oils are sold under various names.

- COLD PRESSED means the oil was squeezed out of the olives by a mechanical press. There is no evidence that this is healthier than other methods of extraction.
- VIRGIN or EXTRA VIRGIN refers to the difference in acid content, not the fat. Oil from the first pressing is often called "extra virgin" and is the most flavourful.
- LIGHT olive oil describes a lighter colour, fragrance or texture.

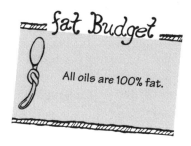

Uncap the cooking magic of different oils

Use oils sparingly and in different ways. In my kitchen you'll find olive oil, which has a wonderful fruity flavour that is delicious on salads. Canola oil is ideal when I need a cooking oil that has no taste. In the fridge is sesame oil which has an intense nutty flavour—so I only need to use a little as a flavouring. Try it on stir-fries.

The name "canola" comes from CANadian Oil, Low Acid.

Margarine and butter

What's the wiser spread for your bread? Both have the same total fat content and therefore the same number of calories, but . . .

Butter contains cholesterol—it comes from an animal source. Margarine is cholesterol-free—it's made from vegetable oils, a plant source.

Both hydrogenated margarine and butter are high in saturated fat. What's more, during processing some of the fat in hydrogenated margarine turns into trans fatty acids. Both of these fats tend to raise cholesterol.

The wise choice? Non-hydrogenated margarine. It has no cholesterol or trans fats and is low in saturated fat.

Fat Budget

1 tsp butter or margarine = 1 tsp fat.

HeartSmart Tip

Choosing margarine?

- Choose a margarine that is non-hydrogenated.
- The softer the margarine, the better.
- Read the label on "light" margarines. They usually contain half the fat. Their water content makes them unsuitable for cooking—and they make toast soggy—but they're ideal for sandwiches or on baked or in mashed potatoes.

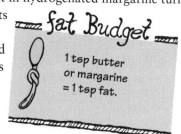

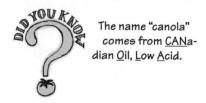

ALL STAR TIP

Palm oil added in small amounts to non-hydrogenated margarine makes the margarine spreadable without creating trans fats.

fat Budget

Choose a light margarine which has half the fat compared to regular margarine.

Cream cheese lovers, rejoice

Compared to butter or margarine, cream cheese has one-third as much fat so it's a good choice—provided you don't use three times as much! You'll find some wonderful tasty new choices on the market flavoured with smoked salmon, garlic or fruit. Look for new lower-fat cream cheeses which have about half the fat. No, you can't count it as a milk serving.

fat Budget

1 tbsp cream cheese = 1 tsp fat.

Salad dressings and mayonnaise

Most of us are looking for lower-fat products and manufacturers have responded. Browse the shelves and you'll come upon lots of low-fat or fat-free salad dressing and mayonnaise. Check the label to find out how many grams of fat each one contains—and zero in on the one with the least.

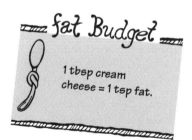

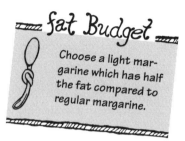

- If it says "low calorie" on the label, a salad dressing is low fat too. The calories in a dressing all come from fat.

ALL STAR TIP

- Make the lunchtime sandwich a variety show. Try other spreads such as salsa, mustard, chutney, cranberry sauce, ketchup or relish. If you're using mayonnaise, skip the margarine or butter.
- Checked the vinegar section recently? What a choice! Red wine, white wine and herb-flavoured vinegars. Balsamic and apple cider vinegar. Raspberry and strawberry vinegar. All waiting to add impact to salads, sauces—even desserts. Make your own in the summer months when berries are ripe and fresh herbs are plentiful.

For flavour's sake, be a little saucy

Borrow ideas from other cuisines around the world and use high-powered sauces for instant flavour. Try teriyaki, hoisin, plum and fiery chili sauce from Asia. Experiment with Mexican salsa or British Worcestershire sauce. While low in fat, some of these sauces may be higher in salt. Use just a touch—that's all you need.

fun food...fast

Dazzling dressings

Creamy Homemade Dressings

Be creative! Blend low-fat yogurt or soft yogurt cheese with a little low-fat mayonnaise. Season with fresh herbs, a minced clove of garlic, fresh basil, dill, oregano, black pepper or chili powder.

Great Vinaigrette Varieties

Mix 2 parts oil—or try even less (see below)—with 1 part vinegar and your favourite herbs. For variety, try red wine vinegar, rice vinegar, balsamic vinegar or raspberry vinegar.

Balsamic Orange Vinaigrette

1/3 cup (75 mL) orange juice
2 tbsp (30 mL) balsamic vinegar
2 tbsp (30 mL) olive oil
1 tsp (5 mL) dry mustard
1/4 cup (50 mL) water
2 tsp (10 mL) chopped parsley

Combine and whisk. Refrigerate for a few hours. Serve with mild-flavoured greens—25 calories and 2 grams fat per 1 tbsp serving.

Keep an eye on your salt intake!

Don't rely on salt for flavour. Here are some easy ways to cut down.

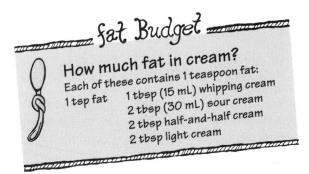

- Be aware of the salt you add when you're cooking and eating. Try taping over half the holes in the salt shaker.
- Use more fresh foods such as homemade soups rather than canned.
- Try spices and seasonings instead of salt. Lemon, mustard powder, garlic, ginger, curry, thyme, parsley or paprika can all lift a dish from bland to mind-blowing.
- Making your own stock and bouillon will let you cut down on the salt and the fat.
- Read labels on processed foods and choose low-salt products whenever possible.
- If you're using a salt substitute, check with your doctor.
- If you have high blood pressure, reduce your salt intake.

Sea salt or table salt: any difference?

Although unrefined sea salt may contain small amounts of some minerals, once refined it's almost the same as ordinary salt, but without the benefit of being iodized.

HeartSmart Tip

Low sodium means a product:

- contains 50% less sodium than the regular product
- contains no more than 40 mg of sodium per 100 g
- has no added salt.

Cream—sweet or sour, it's sinful

There's something unique about the flavour and silkiness of cream. Too bad it's high in fat. See how it fits into your fat budget before you indulge.

fat Budget

How much fat in cream?

Each of these contains 1 teaspoon fat:

1 tsp fat	1 tbsp (15 mL) whipping cream
	2 tbsp (30 mL) sour cream
	2 tbsp half-and-half cream
	2 tbsp light cream

Here's the HeartSmart way to give coffee a stir

Use low-fat milk instead of cream, and skim milk powder instead of coffee whitener.

DID YOU KNOW

Non-dairy coffee whiteners may be cholesterol free but they're not fat free. Often the vegetable oil is hydrogenated or the oil used is palm or coconut oil—high in saturated fat. Many brands have more calories per serving than light cream. A far better buy is skim milk powder.

fat Budget

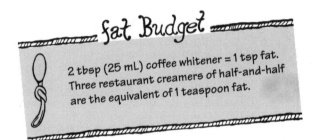

2 tbsp (25 mL) coffee whitener = 1 tsp fat. Three restaurant creamers of half-and-half are the equivalent of 1 teaspoon fat.

ALL STAR TIP

When a recipe calls for sour cream, use low-fat or nonfat versions, or try low-fat yogurt cheese instead. See page 72.

Watch out for invisible fat

Snack foods can hide fat—often too much and often saturated. Cut back on high-fat processed foods. Read labels and try to choose products with the least fat per serving. Go slow as you add these to the #3 part of your cart.

HeartSmart Tip Snack counterattack

- Keep your fridge stocked with fresh veggies and fruit for quick and delicious low-fat snacks.
- Buy lower-fat snacks such as pretzels and plain popcorn rather than chips or nuts.
- Choose sherbet, frozen yogurt or low-fat dairy desserts more often than ice cream.
- Choose cookies and crackers with less than 1 teaspoon fat per serving.

Potato chips, corn chips, tortilla chips, cheese puffs

In themselves, potatoes and corn are low-fat food. Fry them in oil to make chips and look what happens. Suddenly just a few chips—about 15—add up to 2 teaspoons (10 g) of fat. Not to mention the added salt. Heavy on the fat budget.

ALL STAR TIP

- If you have the urge, keep your eyes open for baked chips that are lower in fat and salt. In a Mexican mood? Serve baked tortilla chips with low-fat salsa rather than high-fat guacamole.
- "Low in saturated fat" on a label doesn't necessarily mean that a snack is low in total fat. Don't be misled and think you can eat more.

Popcorn

Granted, it's simple to make, but packaged microwave popcorn is high in fat. Look for the low-fat varieties. A better idea? Make your own popcorn on top of the stove using minimal oil, or use a hot air popper, and salt sparingly.

ALL STAR TIP

Encourage your family to snack on homemade low-fat popcorn, unsalted pretzels, rice cakes or dry breakfast cereal. See Mighty Simple Snacks, page 114.

Chocolate consumption is on the rise, perhaps because eating chocolate releases serotonin, a brain chemical that makes us feel good. The bad news: a typical plain chocolate bar contains at least 3 tsp fat and is loaded with sugar. Remember, 1 tsp fat = approximately 5 g fat.

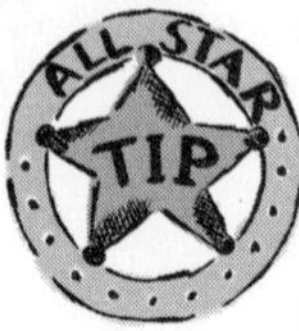

Carob flour is low in fat, but it is combined with coconut oil or hydrogenated vegetable oil for use in chocolate bars so the fat content is as high as chocolate. Whichever way you cut it, carob or chocolate take big bites out of your fat budget.

Dry chocolate-milk powder mixed with skim or 1% milk is a good, lower-fat way to feed that chocolate craving.

fat Budget

Look how popular snacks can attack!

0 tsp fat	1 cup air-popped popcorn
	1 cup pretzels
2 tsp fat	15 chips
3 tsp fat	1 small, plain chocolate bar
7.5 tsp fat	1/2 cup (125 mL) nuts or seeds

Fats, oils and others at a glance

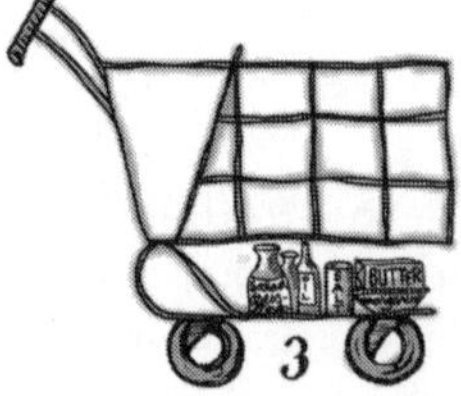

1. Reduce the total quantity of fat in your diet.
2. Think quality. Choose unsaturated fats.
3. Take control of how you spend your fat budget.

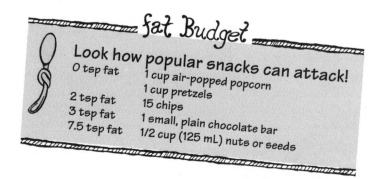

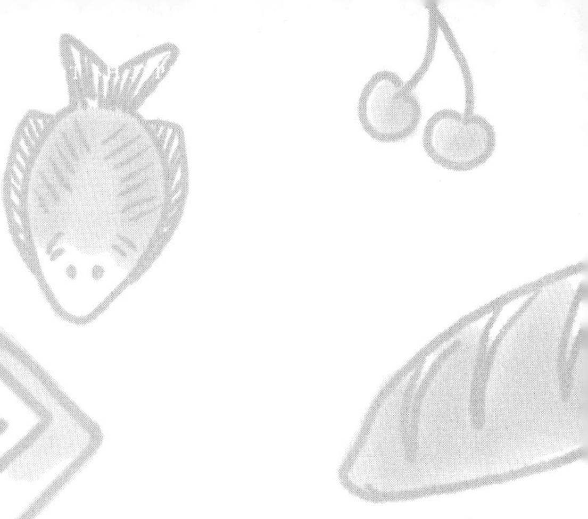

Mighty Meals Mighty Quick

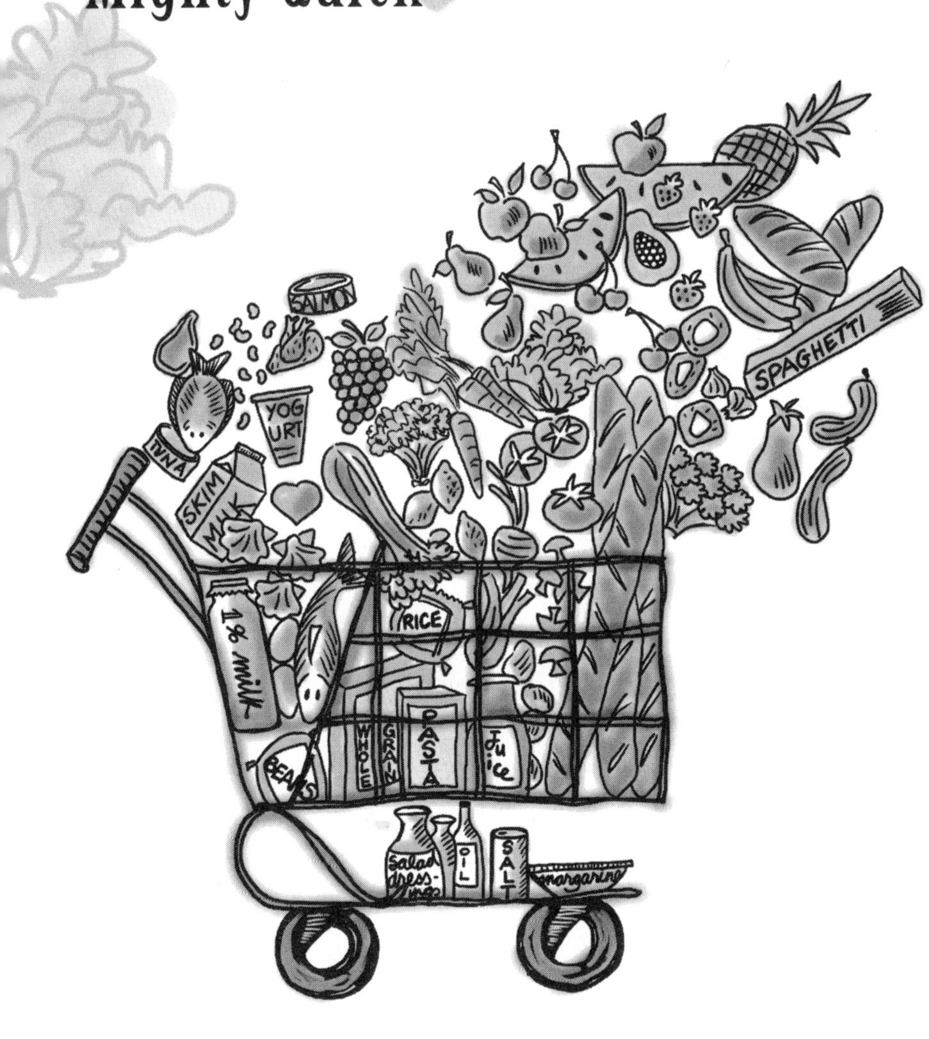

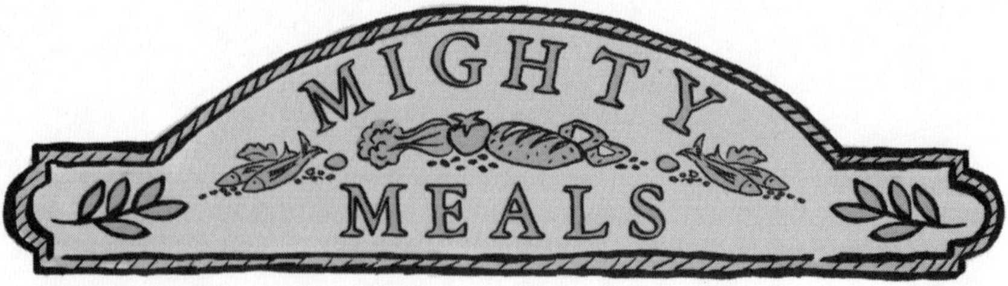

Fill your plate the same way you fill your HeartSmart shopping cart. Load up with grains, fruit and veggies, choose lower-fat meat and milk products and go slow on the fats and oils.

Because I'm a dietitian, people often ask me, "What do you feed your family? Do you ponder over cookbooks all the time? Do you spend hours cooking up a storm?"

To be honest, I have shelves full of tempting books. I love to read them and yes, I love to cook. But I usually only try new recipes when we're entertaining. Sound familiar? On a daily basis, I want no-brainer dishes that are quick, simple, tasty and nutritious. Meals that are mighty in nutrition, that I can make from memory—and that are mighty quick.

We need three meals a day and nutritious snacks. And the better balanced they are, the easier it is to stay well, maintain a healthy weight and control our fat budgets. Breakfast is usually fast and functional. Lunch can be at home or in lunch bags packed with savvy and skill. Supper is loaded with nutrition, and made in minutes.

How to have Mighty Meals every day

These days not many of us have time to follow formal recipes on a daily basis. We need to work with ideas—concepts. These are mine.

As I've shown you throughout this book, fat and nutrient intake are better managed over several days than on a recipe-by-recipe basis. Just follow the concepts and rest assured, they're all HeartSmart.

Beginning with breakfast

The most important meal of the day. Your body hasn't had nourishment in many hours. Your day lies ahead. No wonder you need refuelling. I start every morning with a glass of orange juice, a large bowl of cereal (made from a mix of three different high-fibre cereals) with skim milk and a cup of tea. Fruit, grains and milk—already I've had servings from three of the four bands of the Canada's Food Guide rainbow, and I've chosen a variety of foods from the #1 part of my shopping cart and a lower-fat choice from #2.

One-minute Mighty breakfasts

All of these are nutritious, delicious, low fat—and fast to make.

"Toasted" Cottage Cheese

Spread low-fat cottage cheese on English muffin. Sprinkle with mixture of cinnamon and sugar. Top with sliced bananas or raisins. Broil in toaster oven.

Super Slices

Bagels or whole-wheat toast spread with low-fat cream cheese or peanut butter and jam.

Microwaved Eggs

Mix up 2 beaten eggs in a mug (one whole and one egg white is a lower-fat option). Microwave for 40 seconds at full power and serve with toast.

Power Blender Shake

Blend one cup low-fat milk, a banana, 1 tsp (5 mL) of vanilla and 1 tbsp (15 mL) of honey until frothy. Yum! Other days, add a tablespoon of peanut butter or a half cup (125 mL) of fruit-flavoured low-fat yogurt or fresh fruit.

Two-Minute Lower-cholesterol French Toast (worth that extra minute).

Whisk together 2 egg whites, 2 whole eggs, 1/4 cup (50 mL) low-fat milk, a few drops of vanilla, 2 tsp (10 mL) of sugar, and a pinch of cinnamon. One by one, dip 8 slices of bread into the mixture, coating them well. Lightly grease a nonstick pan and brown on both sides. Makes enough for 4.

Power lunchbags

By the middle of the day many of us are out of the house. It's all too easy to head for the closest fast food joint—and possibly blow our fat budget and our pocketbook for the day. We may even skip lunch. Packing a healthy lunch-bag is easy once you get into the habit, and it's far better nutritionally.

KIDSTUFF

Combat lunchbox trading in your child's schoolyard. Pack lunch together with your kids.

Mighty lunchbag shopping list

Pack a lunch the same way you fill your HeartSmart shopping cart. Load up with whole grains, fruits and veggies. Choose lean meat and low-fat milk products. Be creative with legumes. Go light on the fat you add. Picture a 1-2-3 lunchbag, just like your shopping cart.

ALL STAR TIP

30 minutes of organization = 1-minute lunches

- Tasty sandwich fillings. High-powered fruits and veggies. If you've got them all at hand, you'll use them. A system like this saves you time and money. You just have to be "dedicated."
- DEDICATE one KITCHEN DRAWER for lunch supplies. Here's what goes in it: paper or reusable nylon bags, a thermos, assorted microwaveable plastic containers, drinking bottles, plastic utensils and napkins, a notepad and pen so you can write a quick few lines. Finding a note that says "I love you," or "Hope that exam goes well," will brighten anyone's afternoon.
- DEDICATE one part of the FRIDGE for lunch-only items: yogurt, milk, juice, sandwich fixings (not just the fillings but the mustard and the low-fat mayo). Let your family know that it's hands off for casual snacking.

Build a super sandwich

The Bread

Whole-grain bread, bagels, pitas, buns, submarines, Kaiser buns, dinner rolls or English muffins.

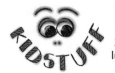

The Spread

A smear, no more, of margarine or butter or mayonnaise (choose the low-fat or fat-free varieties). Mustard, salsa, chutney, cranberry sauce or relish to boost flavour.

The Fillers

Lots of lettuce, tomato, sprouts, cucumber, onions—even sliced oranges. Whatever you have, load up. Layer wet things like tomato between two other fillers and the bread won't go soggy.

The Filling

Lean meats such as turkey breast, low-fat ham or lean beef. Canned salmon or tuna (be light on what you moisten it with). Peanut butter. Chopped hard-cooked egg.

Spread Dijon, honey or other spicy mustard on bread instead of the usual 1 teaspoon of mayo—and save 1 teaspoon of fat.

Plan leftovers for lunch

The lunchroom microwave opens the door to variety. HeartSmart pasta dishes, rice and vegetables, soups and stews can warm you up the next day or can be frozen in lunch-sized portions to make a welcome return appearance later on.

Substantial salads made with beans, grains or pasta also hold up well and make a nice change from sandwiches. So make lots, and make lunch even easier.

Fending off those sneaky snack attacks

Snacking is a national pastime. We all do it. Kids do it whenever they can. Teens do it constantly. But . . . if you keep the fridge and the pantry filled with tasty foods that are low in fat, snacks can be a way to boost everyone's nutrition.

Put fruit juice on your shopping list instead of soft drinks. Keep tubs of yogurt and yogurt-cheese dips in the fridge and a platter of crisp cut-up vegetables right beside them. Buy whole grain breads and crackers, and low-fat cheese instead of cookies and chips.

Mighty simple snacks

- Low-fat milk, cheese and yogurt
- Cereal
- Fresh fruit
- Bagels or pita bread spread thinly with light cream cheese (make your own bagel chips by toasting sliced-up bagels in the oven and dip in salsa)
- Cut veggies prebagged so that they're user-friendly. Serve with low-fat or fat-free salad dressing or low-fat yogurt-cheese dips
- Homemade low-fat muffins
- Mini-pizza on English muffin or pita bread
- Low-fat cheese and crackers
- Unbuttered popcorn—air popped is best. Keep the air-popper on your kitchen counter so it's easy to use. Toss with herbs or spices.
- Low-fat yogurt—look for 1% milk fat or less and mix with cut-up fruit
- Vegetable or tomato juice
- Unsweetened ready-to-eat cereal
- Fruit kebabs—just thread whole strawberries, grapes, banana pieces or orange segments on wooden skewers
- Rice cakes spread thinly with peanut butter, almond butter or light cream cheese
- Frozen juice popsicles or light fudgsicles
- Hummus and pita bread
- Homemade corn chips. Cut tortillas into wedges. Bake in single layer 400°F (200°C) for 8 minutes, or until lightly browned and crisp.

Guess how much sugar there is in a can of pop. A teaspoon? Two? Guess again. A glass of pop contains 7.5 teaspoons of sugar. It's like eating a handful of sugar cubes.

Fruit drink isn't the same as fruit juice. If it doesn't say "juice" on the bottle or package, then it isn't. There may be as little as 10% juice in fruit punch, cocktail or beverage. Your best bet is to buy products labelled "juice" or you may be paying a premium for expensive sugar water! Remember, the ingredient at the top of the list is present in the greatest quantity.

DID YOU KNOW

Have a cuppa...tea or coffee

Despite scores of studies on caffeine, there is no conclusive evidence suggesting that it is harmful. According to Nutrition Recommendations for Canadians, a moderate caffeine intake is four cups a day of drip coffee. (Check the size of your coffee cup—some of the new cups can be as large as two regular cups.) Tea, chocolate, colas and some over-the-counter medications also contain caffeine.

Dinners in a dash

Fill your plate the same way you fill your HeartSmart shopping cart. Be lavish with grains and vegetables. Use meat as an accent. Go slow on the fats and oils. Make the main event a delicious stir-fry, pasta, or soup and salad.

Remember the old saying: "Eat breakfast like a king, lunch like a queen and dinner like a pauper." The last meal of the day can be a lot lighter than we're used to.

Add up all the variations you can create around a few favourites, and you could put a different dinner on the table every night of the year. What's even better? These mighty dishes are so simple they don't even need recipes. Just remember a few easy steps.

Low in fat, high in flavour: six quick tips

Fat carries flavours, which is why we sometimes find it hard to cut back. The trick? Replace it with other intense and satisfying flavours—or let a food's own great, natural taste shine through.

1. Cook rice, beans and grains in stock with added herbs and garlic.
2. Add zest and shine to grilled foods with mustards, jams and chutneys.
3. Use nonstick cookware so you need less cooking fat.
4. Substitute oil with stock, juice or wine to moisten and baste meats.
5. Use a spray bottle filled with oil to lightly dress a salad.
6. Add herbs and spices. They're terrific flavour boosters that let you limit fat and salt. Feel free to experiment.

ALL STAR TIP

Ground spices lose their flavour quickly. Buy a little at a time—or buy them whole and grind as needed. Store them in a cool, dry place.

ALL STAR TIP

- Before you add fresh herbs to a dish, rub them between your hands to release their flavour.
- Increase the flavour of spices (but not dried herbs) by heating them in a dry pan until just fragrant.

PENNYWISE

Got a sunny window in your kitchen? It's the perfect spot for a few containers of fresh herbs. That way you'll get used to snipping them to add to soups and savoury dishes—with sparkling results. Fresh basil with tomatoes is a magical combination. Oregano or savory really wake up green beans. French and Italian herbs—rosemary, thyme, marjoram and sage—all add flair to pastas, vegetables and casseroles.

Q

What about frozen dinners?

A

You can't beat them for convenience, but you can often beat them for nutrition. Reading the labels is the easiest way to decide if you want to add them to your shopping cart. Look for lean entrees and meats that are lower in fat and calories. Remember, the ingredients at the top of the list are there in the greatest quantity.

"Light": may mean less food, but not necessarily less fat, sugar and salt.

Fat: look for dinners with less than 30% calories from fat.

Salt: look for products with as little as possible. You can always bump up flavour by adding lemon juice or herbs.

ALL STAR TIP

Make your own frozen TV dinners. Buy compartmentalized freezable, microwaveable containers and use them for leftovers—planned or unplanned.

Pasta power

Long skinny spaghetti, linguine and fettuccini. Spirals, shells and pasta shaped like little ears. You'll find at least one for every day of the month!

Add pasta to a big pot of boiling water—skip the salt. Boil dried pasta uncovered, stirring occasionally, until tender but firm, about 12 minutes. Drain immediately in colander (there's no need to rinse), toss with sauce and serve.

Sensationally simple sauces

Quick Tomato Sauce

Sauté chopped onion and garlic in broth or a teaspoon of olive oil. Add a can of plum tomatoes (break them up with a wooden spoon). Simmer for 30 minutes. Add dried or fresh basil and season to taste. Hint: make lots and freeze the leftovers, or use a tomato-based bought sauce.

Variations

Add chopped fresh vegetables such as peppers, mushrooms or zucchini. Throw in a handful of frozen peas—or any other frozen vegetable. Stir in a drained can of tuna. Add scallops for a special treat. Leftover cubed chicken can go in at the last minute so it just warms through.

Top with parmesan cheese and freshly ground pepper. Serve with salad and French bread.

DID YOU KNOW

One tablespoon (15 mL) of grated parmesan has only 2 grams fat and 25 calories, but it is fairly high in sodium.

ALL STAR TIP

Match pasta shapes to pasta sauces

- Hollow pastas (elbows, shells, rigatoni): let them trap thick, chunky sauces.
- Wide pasta (fettuccini): mix with creamy sauces.
- Long pasta (spaghetti or linguine): tomato or seafood sauces.
- Small pasta shapes (orzo and alphabet noodles): use in soups.
- Fresh pasta: light tomato-based sauces—they absorb more liquid than dried pasta.

Stir-fry suppers

Stir-fries are a deceptively simple way to create a host of different dishes, to make the most of a little meat and to enjoy a bounty of tender-crisp vegetables.

Stir-fry suppers

Preheat your wok or nonstick pan. Add a smidgen of oil and swirl around to coat the surface. You'll need less oil provided it's hot enough when you cook the veggies. Even better, use stock or try low-fat salad dressings. Add chopped garlic and ginger and stir-fry for a few seconds.

Add veggies—cut them ahead of time (or use up those snacking vegetables that have been in the fridge for a day or two). Start with those that take longest to cook such as onions, broccoli or cauliflower. End with snow peas or mushrooms that cook in a wink. My favourite combo bursts with colour and texture: mushrooms, broccoli, red and green pepper, chickpeas, zucchini, canned baby corn. Make the palette on your plate a delight to your palate.

For variety, introduce the meat and alternatives group. Sliced lean beef, chunks of chicken breast, tofu or scallops. Stir-fry these before you cook the vegetables. Keep warm on a plate, then add when vegetables are tender.

Wake up your tastebuds with something different. Add chunks of pineapple or apple.

Push stir-fried ingredients to sides of wok or frying pan and add zing to your stir-fry with sauce. Cook until thickened. Here are some of my favourites.

Basic Sauce

2 tsp (10 mL) cornstarch	1 tbsp (15 mL) water
1/2 cup (125 mL) stock	2 tsp (10 mL) light soy sauce
2 tsp (10 mL) honey	1/4 tsp (1 mL) garlic powder

Mix cornstarch with water until smooth. Add other ingredients.

Variations

- SWEET AND SOUR: use pineapple juice instead of chicken stock—a bonus, it's lower in salt. Toss in some pineapple pieces and stir-fry. Yum.
- SZECHUAN SPICY SAUCE: use chili oil in place of cooking oil and add a pinch of dried chili peppers to the basic sauce.

- THAI SAUCE: add 2 tbsp (25 mL) hoisin sauce, 2 tsp (10 mL) each of sesame oil and rice vinegar and 1 tsp (5 mL) dry mustard instead of the soy sauce and honey.

Sprinkle a few toasted peanuts, cashews, sesame seeds or almonds over your stir-fry. Go lightly, these contain fat. Serve with steamed rice (see page 36) and whole-wheat rolls.

Super chicken

You can't beat chicken for versatility. Choose breasts, remove the skin and go dippin' for flavour.

Amazin' chicken dippin'

Remove skin from chicken breasts. Allow one half per person. Season it sensationally. Combine and pour over chicken one of the following:

- Equal amounts of low-fat Italian or Russian dressing mixed with plum or apricot jam. Onion soup mix contributes a wonderful flavour but it does add salt.
- Combine 2 tbsp (25 mL) each Worcestershire sauce, vinegar and chutney, 2 1/2 tbsp (35 mL) ketchup and a chopped green onion, and marinate for 30 minutes.
- Mix 1/4 cup lemon juice, 2 tsp (10 mL) oil, 2 tsp (10 mL) prepared mustard and marinate.
- Spread chicken generously with Dijon mustard and toss in bag of breadcrumbs until coated. Amazingly simple. Outstandingly good.

Bake uncovered at 350°F (180°C) for one hour.

Serve with low-fat french "fries" (page 56) cooked alongside, and a stir-fry of zucchini and tomatoes seasoned with basil, garlic and parsley. Check out Veggie power (page 54). Green salad on the side.

Fish made fabulous

Plain, simple fish is the perfect low-fat choice for a healthy meal. Bake, broil or grill, adding flavor with herbs, citrus juice or spicy salsas.

Wash white fish such as cod, halibut or sole. Pat dry with a paper towel and place in a single layer in a lightly greased casserole.

A world of fish

- Go Mexican and cover with salsa—Spanish for "sauce."
- For Chinese seasoning add fresh ginger, lower-salt soy sauce and scallions.
- Enjoy Japanese teriyaki by marinating in a mixture of 2 tbsp (25 mL) Dijon mustard, 3 tbsp (50 mL) brown sugar, 2 tbsp (25 mL) lower-salt soy sauce, 1 tsp (5 mL) sesame oil and 1 tsp (5 mL) sesame seeds. A sensation.
- Marinate fish for 10 minutes in a commercial marinade or your own made from a finely chopped tomato and red pepper, 1 tbsp (15 mL) each of olive oil and balsamic vinegar and a big pinch of basil, either dried or fresh.
- Pour a can of creamed, low-salt canned soup (mushroom or celery) over the fish.

Add chopped or sliced vegetables and bake uncovered at 350°F (180°C)—or bake the fish on top of the veggies and baste frequently. Bake fish 10 minutes for every inch of thickness.

Serve with rice (page 37), pasta or potatoes and a green salad.

Low-fat Breaded Fish Sticks

Go double dipping with filleted strips of fish:

- Dip in a mixture of low-fat milk and egg white.
- Then dip in dry breadcrumbs seasoned with thyme, basil or dill.
- Line baking sheet with foil, spray with nonstick cooking spray and layer with fish sticks. Bake at 400°F (210°C) for 10 minutes.

Meat marvels

Switch gears on meat—consider it an accent rather than the main course. Choose lean meat, trim external fat and marinate to tenderize.

Meat that s-t-r-e-t-c-h-e-s

Remember, a serving is the size of a deck of cards. Make your meat s-t-r-e-t-c-h. Here's how.

Kebabs

Alternate cubes of marinated lean meat or poultry with cubed green peppers, whole cherry tomatoes, mushrooms and pineapple pieces or apricot halves. Broil or grill 3-5 minutes each side. Serve with rice and large salad.

Fajitas

In nonstick frying pan or wok, sauté lean meat in 2 tsp oil or stock until cooked. Set aside. Saute onions and peppers until tender. Add meat and heat through. Season to taste. Spread hoisin sauce on warmed flour tortillas (wrap in foil and heat at 350°F [180°C] for about 8 minutes), cover with meat and vegetable mixture, shredded lettuce and diced tomato. Roll and enjoy.

Let your family create their personalized fajitas—try roasted vegetables, salsa or non-fat yogurt as toppings, pita bread instead of tortillas, and chicken in place of meat.

Stir-fries

Add thinly sliced meat to your mound of vegetables. Serve on a bed of rice or pasta.

M-m-m-marinades

Lean meat doesn't have to be tough and dry. Marinating it for 4-8 hours in wine or vinegar will make it meltingly tender and flavourful. Here's my favourite:

Chop an onion, mince a garlic clove and grate a chunk of fresh ginger. Add 2 tbsp (30 mL) each of brown sugar, lemon juice, ketchup, Worcestershire sauce and oil and mix in 1/2 cup (125 mL) lower-salt soy sauce. Marinate lean meat overnight in the mixture. Barbecue or grill for 3 to 5 minutes on each side. Slice thinly on the diagonal.

Souper soups

Shout it out … this is one of the best-kept nutrition secrets in town. Soup can be low in calories, high in fibre and loaded with nutrients. Want some examples?

Please sir—may I have some more?

Chicken Soup to Build On

Best the next day—it's worth the wait.

Cover chicken parts with 4 litres of cold water. Use breasts if you want to eat the chicken, economical backs and necks if you just want the flavour. Bring to a boil and skim. Add sliced vegetables—onions, carrots, celery stalks with their leaves, a skinned tomato and a parsnip. Season with 1/2 tsp (2 mL) thyme, 1 bay leaf, 4 cloves garlic, 6 peppercorns, salt and pepper to taste. Simmer for about two hours. Place in fridge overnight and remove the fat that settles on the top.

Make enough soup and you can enjoy it several ways: enjoy as is; add noodles, macaroni or rice; or strain and concentrate to make a handy chicken stock for cooking.

Serve with whole-grain buns and a green salad. Fresh fruit is a nice note to end on.

Bean and Barley Soup

Most people have a favourite recipe from mom. This is one of mine.

Bring 4 litres stock to a boil. Add 1 cup (250 mL) barley, washed and drained, and 1 cup (250 mL) large dried lima beans. Chop and add celery, onion and carrots. Season with a pinch of thyme, basil and ground pepper.

Cook slowly for 1 to 1 1/2 hours until beans are tender. If too thick, add water.

For a delicious meatless thick pea soup, use 2 cups (500 mL) dried green split peas instead of beans and barley

Serve soup with warmed whole-grain buns and a green salad. Delight the family with yogurt-topped baked apples for dessert.

Marvelous Italian Minestrone.

Add a cornucopia of seasonal vegetables to gently simmering broth. The longest-cooking ones—potatoes, carrots, onions—go in first. The fastest-cooking kinds—leeks, green beans, zucchini—go in last. Boost your nutrition by adding pasta, beans or rice. Use your biggest soup pot. Minestrone tastes even better reheated—and it freezes beautifully.

Soup "cans" to remember

ALL STAR TIP

- You *can* do away with added oil, butter or margarine, even if a recipe calls for it. Try it without and see if you notice any difference.
- You *can* still enjoy creamed and thickened soups the Heart-Smart way. Thicken them with potatoes, beans, noodles, rice or pureed vegetables, or use low-fat milk.
- You *can* easily make your own stock and control its salt and fat content. To make handy stock "cubes" for cooking, boil broth down to concentrate flavour. Strain. Freeze in ice cube trays.
- *Canned* broth may contain fat and salt. To remove fat, refrigerate the can so that the fat solidifies on the surface. Look for low-salt varieties.

Pizza pleasures

Keep the basics in your kitchen and you can put together a terrific pizza faster than it takes to order out. It's a lot cheaper too. Keep an eye on the amount of fat you add by using smaller quantities of lower-fat mozzarella cheese, avoiding high-fat meat choices and choosing lower-fat pizza shells.

Pizza with pizzaz

For the base, use pita bread or packaged whole-wheat pizza shells. Choose the mini-pitas and let your family build custom pizzas. Spread with bottled or homemade tomato sauce (see page 36). Top with vegetables—almost anything goes. Sliced tomatoes, mushrooms or peppers, artichoke hearts, broccoli florets, minced sun-dried tomatoes, roasted vegetables (see page 55). Highlight with a sprinkling of chopped olives, capers or anchovies.

Sprinkle lightly with lower-fat mozzarella cheese.

Add freshly ground pepper plus a sprinkling of dried basil or rosemary. Bake in hot oven for 10 minutes. Enjoy a big green salad on the side.

The End!

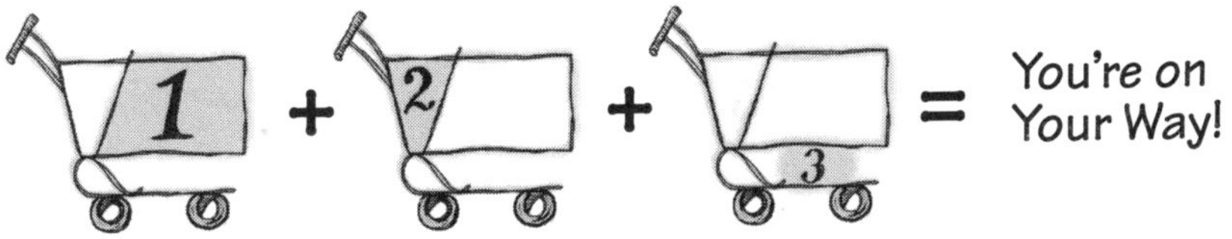

Appendix

Where foods fit in the total nutrition picture

CANADA'S FOOD GUIDE TO HEALTHY EATING	GRAIN PRODUCTS	VEGETABLES & FRUIT	MILK PRODUCTS	MEAT & ALTERNATIVES
PROTEIN	Protein	—	Protein	Protein
FAT	—	—	Fat	Fat
CARBOHYDRATE	Carbohydrate	Carbohydrate	Carbohydrate	—
FIBRE	Fibre	Fibre	—	—
VITAMINS				
Thiamin	Thiamin	Thiamin	—	Thiamin
Riboflavin	Riboflavin	—	Riboflavin	Riboflavin
Niacin	Niacin	—	—	Niacin
Folacin	Folacin	Folacin	—	Folacin
Vitamin B12	—	—	Vitamin B12	Vitamin B12
Vitamin C	—	Vitamin C	—	—
Vitamin A	—	Vitamin A	Vitamin A	—
Vitamin D	—	—	Vitamin D	—
Calcium	—	—	Calcium	—
MINERALS				
Iron	Iron	Iron	—	Iron
Zinc	Zinc	—	Zinc	Zinc
Magnesium	Magnesium	Magnesium	Magnesium	Magnesium

Source: Using the Food Guide, Health and Welfare Canada, 1992

My Four Steps to Estimating Your Personal Fat Budget

I use these four simple steps to determine an individual's personal fat budget. Try it!

1. Find your desirable body weight by using the range in the B.M.I. chart (below):
Desirable body weight = __________ kg

2. Calculate how many calories you need by multiplying your desirable weight by your activity factor:
If you are sedentary, multiply your desirable weight by 30.
If you are moderately active, multiply your desirable weight by 35.
If you are *very* active, multiply your desirable weight by 40.
Desirable body weight _________ kg X _________ = ________ calories

3. Calculate your fat budget in grams:
Divide the calories needed per day (Step 2) by 30.
________ calories ÷ 30 = ________ grams of fat

4. Calculate your fat budget in teaspoons:
Divide your fat budget grams (Step 3) by 5.
________ grams of fat ÷ 5 = ________ teaspoons of fat

Your Personal Fat Budget is ________ *teaspoons of fat per day.*

Body Mass Index Chart

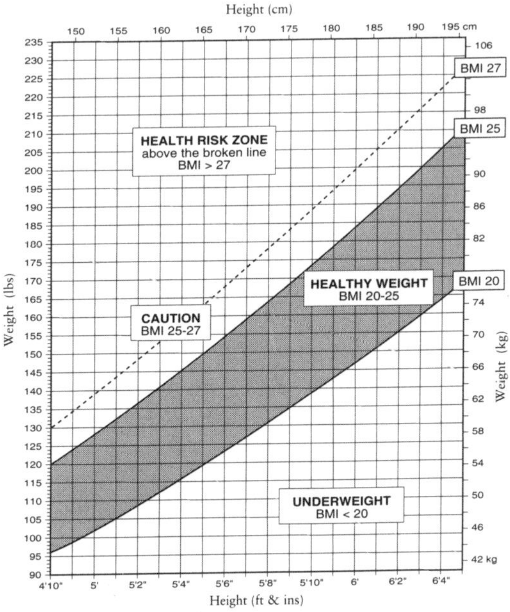

Source:
Nutrition Services,
Ottawa–Carleton Health
Department, 1987

Fats and heart health

SATURATED FATS: tend to raise blood cholesterol. Usually solid at room temperature. Reduce your intake of these fats.

Key sources: meat, poultry, milk products (except skim-milk products), butter, lard, tropical oils (palm, palm kernel and coconut) which are found in foods such as baked goods and other convenience foods.

MONOUNSATURATED FATS: help to lower blood cholesterol. Usually liquid at room temperature.

Key sources: olive oil, canola oil, avocado, olives, nuts such as almonds, pistachios, pecans, hazelnuts and cashews.

POLYUNSATURATED FATS: help to lower blood cholesterol. Usually liquid at room temperature, they contain essential fatty acids which your body cannot manufacture.

Key sources: vegetable oils like safflower, sunflower, corn, soybean and most nut oils, nuts such as walnuts, pine nuts, brazil nuts and chestnuts, sunflower seeds, sesame seeds and fish.

OMEGA-3 FATTY ACIDS: a group of polyunsaturated fats. May help to lessen the risk of heart disease and stroke by reducing blood clotting and making platelets less likely to stick together.

Key sources: fatty fish such as salmon, trout and mackerel; canola, soy and flax oils.

HYDROGENATION: a process in which hydrogen is added to liquid vegetable oil changing it into a solid, which is more saturated and has a longer shelf life.

Key sources: vegetable shortening and other foods made with vegetable shortening such as cookies, crackers, chips and other packaged foods, some peanut butter and many but not all margarines.

TRANS FATTY ACIDS: created during the process of hydrogenation. They have been shown to raise blood cholesterol levels. Technically unsaturated fats, they act more like saturated fats.

Key sources: vegetable shortening and other foods made with vegetable shortening such as cookies, crackers, chips and other packaged foods, some peanut butter and many but not all margarines.

Figuring out the percentage of fat in a food

To calculate how many calories in a food come from fat:

1. Multiply the number of grams of fat by 9 (1 gram = 9 calories)—if a serving has 5 grams of fat, then 45 calories come from fat.
2. Divide the result by the number of calories in the serving. If the total calories of the serving are 90, then 45 ÷ 90 = 0.5 calories from fat.
3. Multiply the number by 100 to get the percentage—0.5 x 100 = 50% calories from fat.

Remember:

1. The 30% figure applies to your overall diet—what you eat over a day or a week. You don't need to figure it out for every individual food.
2. The percentage of fat calories is not as important if you eat the foods very rarely or if you don't eat much.
3. The percentage of fat calories is not as important when the food is low in calories.

Sources of cholesterol

Health and Welfare Canada—Nutrition Recommendations 1990 suggests that "reducing the cholesterol intake of the population towards 300 mg/day or less would be beneficial in the long term for the reduction of mortality from coronary artery disease."

Here are some common sources of dietary cholesterol. Remember, cholesterol is found only in foods from animals and fish.

mg cholesterol	quantity	
70-120	3.5 oz (100 g)	beef, pork, lamb, most cuts
75-100	"	poultry
432	"	eggs, 2 large
415	"	beef liver
631	"	chicken liver
344	"	kidney
53	"	clams
48	"	scallops
45	"	oysters
87	"	crab
78	"	lobster

125-160	3.5 oz (100 g) shrimp
10	1 cup (250 mL) milk, 1% fat
35	1 cup (250 mL) milk, whole
31	1 tablespoon (15 mL) butter
47	1.5 oz (45 g) cheddar cheese

Nutrition claims

Canadian consumers are protected by legislation. Health Canada is reviewing the rules as we go to press, but until the changes are announced, these are the definitions.

1. Calorie claims

What it says	What it means
Calorie-reduced	Contains 50% fewer calories than the same food when not calorie-reduced
Low calorie	Contains 15 calories or less per serving. Contains fewer calories than a calorie-reduced food but more than a calorie-free food
Calorie free	Contains no more than 1 calorie per 100 g
Source of energy	Contains at least 100 calories per serving (see label for serving size)

2. Fat claims

What it says	What it means
Low in fat	No more than 3 g fat per serving
Fat free	No more than 0.5 g fat per 100 g (approved by Health Canada, May 1997)
Reduced in fat	Must contain at least 25% less fat and at least 1.5 g less fat per serving than the regular product
Low in cholesterol	No more than 20 mg cholesterol per serving and per 100 g
Cholesterol free	No more than 3 mg cholesterol per serving

3. Sugar claims

What it says	What it means
Low in sugar	Contains no more than 2 g sugar per serving
No sugar added, or unsweetened	Has no sugar added during processing although it may contain naturally present sugar
Sugar free	Contains no more than 0.25 g sugar per 100 g and no more than 1 calorie per 100 g.

4. Dietary fibre claims

What it says	What it means
Source of dietary fibre	At least 2 g dietary fibre per serving
High source	At least 4 g dietary fibre per serving
Very high source	At least 6 g dietary fibre per serving

5. Salt and sodium claims

What it says	What it means
Low sodium or low salt	Contains 50% less sodium than the regular product and not more than 40 mg sodium per 100 g (exceptions: cheddar cheese may contain up to 50 mg of sodium per 100 g; meat, poultry and fish may contain up to 80 mg of sodium per 100 g)
No added salt or unsalted	No salt is added to the food and none of the ingredients contain a large quantity of salt
Salt free or sodium free	No more than 5 mg sodium per 100 g

Sources of dietary fibre

Very high source

More than 6 g/serving

1/3 cup (75 mL)	some all-bran cereals (check label)
1/2 cup (125 mL)	baked beans in tomato sauce
1/2 cup (125 mL)	kidney beans

High source

More than 4 g/serving

2/3 cup (150 mL)	some bran cereals (check label)
1/4 cup (50 mL)	100% wheat bran
1/2 cup (125 mL)	dried peas, lima beans, navy beans
1 cup	wild rice

Source

More than 2 g/serving

1/2 cup (125 mL)	some bran cereals (check label)
1/4 cup (50 mL)	wheat germ
2 slices	whole wheat bread
1/2 cup (125 mL)	lentils
1 cup (250 mL)	brown rice
1/2 cup (125 mL)	corn, peas, spinach, brussels sprouts
1 medium	potato with skin
1/2 cup (125 mL)	berries and cantaloupe
1/2 medium	pear
1 medium	apple, banana, orange, broccoli, carrots
2	prunes
3 tbsp (50 mL)	raisins

Heart-Healthy Cookbooks
from the Heart and Stroke Foundation of Canada

The Light-Hearted Cookbook by Anne Lindsay (MacMillan of Canada)

Lighthearted Everyday Cooking by Anne Lindsay (MacMillan of Canada)

Simply HeartSmart Cooking by Bonnie Stern (Random House of Canada)

More HeartSmart Cooking by Bonnie Stern (Random House of Canada)

HeartSmart Chinese Cooking by Stephen Wong (Douglas & McIntyre)

Index